# Bacterial **Skin Infections** in Small Animals

Plaza Antonio Beltrán Martínez nº 1, planta 8 - letra I
(Centro empresarial El Trovador)
50002 Zaragoza - Spain

First printing: August 2019

This book was originally published in Spanish under the title:
*Infecciones cutáneas bacterianas en pequeños animales*
© 2019 Grupo Asís Biomedia, SL
ISBN Spanish edition: 978-84-17640-06-4

Translation:
Owen Howard

ISBN: 978-84-17640-69-9
DL: Z 1501-2019

Design, layout and printing:
Servet editorial - Grupo Asís Biomedia, SL
www.grupoasis.com
info@grupoasis.com

GRUPO asis

**Servet is the publishing house of Grupo Asís**



Warning:

Veterinary science is constantly evolving, as are pharmacology and the other sciences. Inevitably, it is therefore the responsibility of the veterinary surgeon to determine and verify the dosage, the method of administration, the duration of treatment and any possible contraindications to the treatments given to each individual patient, based on his or her professional experience. Neither the publisher nor the author can be held liable for any damage or harm caused to people, animals or properties resulting from the correct or incorrect application of the information contained in this book.

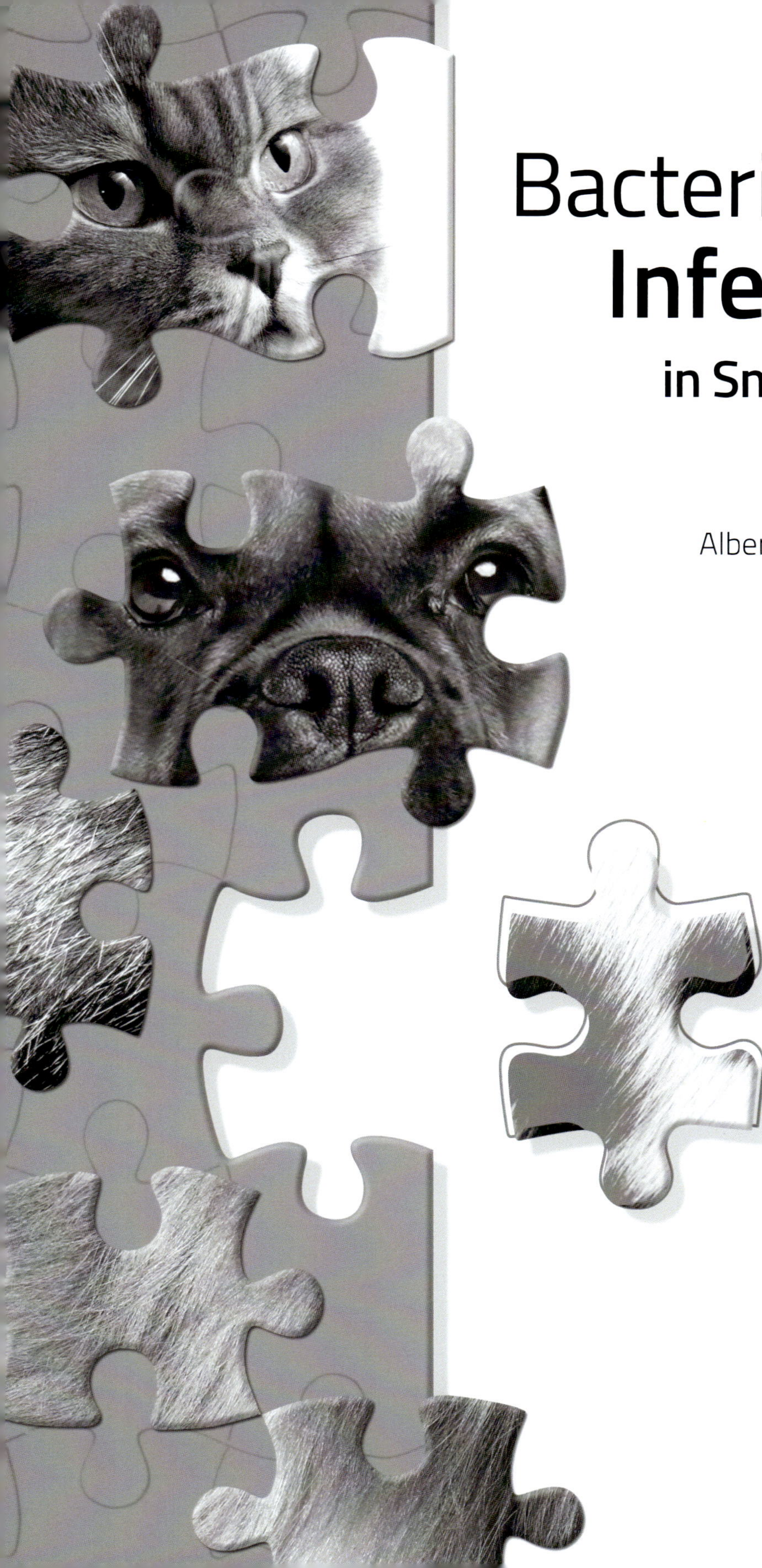

# Bacterial Skin **Infections** in Small Animals

Alberto Martin Cordero

SERVET

*This book is dedicated to my parents Iliana and Alberto,*
*for always supporting me in my studies;*
*to Zuzu, my sister and childhood companion;*
*and my wife Gloria and my son Santiago,*
*who provide me with my motivation.*

# THE AUTHOR

## Alberto Martin Cordero

Dr Alberto Martin Cordero holds a degree in veterinary medicine from the University of Guadalajara (Jalisco, Mexico) and received his postgraduate degree in veterinary dermatology from the European School for Advanced Veterinary Studies at the University of Luxembourg. He has participated in training courses at the NAVC Institute in Florida (USA) and has been a visiting researcher at Animal Dermatology Clinics (California, USA), Colorado State University (USA), and Ludwig Maximilian University (Munich, Germany). He is a de facto diplomate of the Latin American College of Veterinary Dermatology.

He currently works in private practice and is the owner of Vetderm: Dermatología Veterinaria Especializada (Specialised Veterinary Dermatology), the first veterinary referral clinic specialising in dermatology in Guadalajara (Mexico). He is also a professor at the Department of Veterinary Medicine of the University of Guadalajara.

He is a member of the Programming Committee of the North American Veterinary Dermatology Forum (NAVDF), a founding member of the Latin American Society of Veterinary Dermatology (SLDV), and a Veterinary Dermatology Coordinator for the Veterinary Congress of León (Mexico).

His main interests are diseases of the ears of dogs and cats, as well as allergic diseases of the skin and video otoscopy.

He has published several articles and clinical cases in national and international journals, and has presented at congresses in Mexico, Central America, South America, Eastern Europe, and Asia.

# FOREWORD

Alberto Martin Cordero is a veterinary surgeon with a deep passion for veterinary dermatology. I feel honoured to write the preface to this wonderful book.

I believe it is important that the reader knows a little, both personally and professionally, about the author of the book they are about to read. Alberto's passions are evident in many aspects of his life. He is passionate about sharing knowledge, and gives courses, workshops, and talks in various fields and countries, publishes articles in renowned journals, and is continually working on research projects. He has great desire to further expand the field of veterinary dermatology, thereby creating new opportunities for other professionals. His passions are not limited to the professional sphere: comics, superhero movies, and fantasy are part of his personality, and all make appearances in his talks and presentations. In addition to the above, Alberto is an exemplary husband and a dedicated father who is always present in his son's life.

In this, his second book, he focuses on bacterial infections in veterinary dermatology, specifically those affecting dogs. This book is particularly timely, given the increasing prevalence of bacterial resistance to antibiotics and the consequent changes that this has necessitated in the treatment of skin infections. Today more than ever, knowledge of basic concepts relating to the treatment of bacterial infections is an essential requirement for the clinical veterinary surgeon: how to correctly diagnose bacterial infections, how and when to perform bacterial cultures and antibiotic sensitivity tests and interpret the results obtained, the treatment implications of a biofilm,  how to administer topical therapy, or how to replace systemic antibiotics with local, topical therapy.

Veterinary surgeons have a responsibility to care for the health of their patients, but also play a very important role in the health of humans who live with pets, since they must diagnose and correctly treat infections with great zoonotic potential, and safeguard the useful life of antibiotics. It is up to us to make the relevant changes in antibiotic use and to prescribe them in the most effective and prudent way. I have no doubt that readers will greatly benefit from this practical and dynamic book, which presents the most up-to-date and relevant veterinary information relating to clinical dermatology in dogs and cats.

**Galia Sheinberg W.**

MVZ, Esp. Dermatologist and veterinary allergist

# PREFACE

Writing a book about bacterial skin infections presents many challenges. The main challenge is taking the reader (the clinical veterinary surgeon) beyond the basic concepts taught in university classrooms about bacterial infections. The second challenge is integrating preexisting knowledge with newer concepts such as the equilibrium of the patient's microbiota, a topic that has received considerable research attention of late and will no doubt continue to occupy column inches in medical journals. The third challenge is to accompany the reader on the search for the source of the bacterial skin infection, and to move away from the idea of merely treating the infection itself.

Finally, it is essential to change the prescribing habits of clinical veterinary surgeons and to impress upon them the importance of correct use of antimicrobial agents. This is the most important change required in order to wage an effective war on the problem of growing bacterial resistance. It also poses the greatest challenge, since it requires modification of habits acquired over many years.

This book provides readers with many tools that I hope they will find useful in daily clinical practice, as well as information acquired from numerous publications, dermatology books, and a large number of challenging cases that I have encountered throughout my professional career.

In addition to providing readers with some answers, I hope that this book raises some important questions that can be addressed in the future through studies and publications arising from our daily work with clinical cases that put our skills to the test, but also inspire us to search for new solutions.

**The author, Alberto Martin Cordero**

# TABLE OF CONTENTS

# 01

# THE SKIN MICROBIOME AND DIAGNOSIS OF BACTERIAL SKIN INFECTIONS

## The skin microbiome and skin infections

### Microbiome and microbiota

Since their discovery, bacteria have been largely considered harmful, both within the field of medicine and by the general public. However, recent studies have shown that most bacteria that reside in the different organ systems are beneficial, and live in equilibrium with the different microorganisms with which they cohabitate, preventing the proliferation of specific microorganisms and subsequent infection. These bacteria also compete for nutrients with other potentially pathogenic bacteria, facilitating immune system development and producing numerous metabolites.

In the last 20 years, several studies have revealed the complexity of the communities of microorganisms that inhabit the skin surface of animals and humans. These communities have a commensal (and in some cases codependent) relationship with the host, and help maintain an equilibrium that prevents overgrowth of other microorganisms with pathogenic potential.

Bacteria that normally inhabit certain systems were previously known as bacterial flora. However, in recent years this concept has evolved, and in 2000 Lederberg coined the term microbiome to describe a balanced relationship between humans and microorganisms.

The term microbiome covers a wide range of microorganisms, including bacteria, fungi, viruses, and parasites; their genes and metabolites; and the conditions within their habitats. By contrast, the term microbiota (Table 1) describes a collection of microorganisms in a defined microenvironment. Currently, this term is preferable to microflora, which refers to microscopic plants. Characterisation of the microbiota is often based on the genes found in bacteria and fungi.

Dysbiosis (also known as dysbacteriosis) describes an imbalance of the normal microbiota caused by quantitative or qualitative changes in its composition or changes in its function, metabolic activities, or distribution.

**Table 1.** Diversity of the cutaneous microbiota in dogs, cats, and humans in different sampling sites.

| Host | Cutaneous sites and skin condition | Composition of the microbiota |
|---|---|---|
| **Dog** | Mucosal surface or mucocutaneous junctions | *Proteobacteria*, *Firmicutes*, *Actinobacteria*, and *Bacteroidetes*. *Moraxella* (predominant in nostrils), *Proteobacteria*, and *Bacteroidetes* in the labial commissures |
| | Skin with hair | *Proteobacteria* (more abundant), *Firmicutes*, *Actinobacteria*, and *Bacteroidetes* |
| **Cat** | Normal skin | *Proteobacteria*, *Bacteroidetes*, and *Actinobacteria* (more abundant in oral cavity) |
| **Human** | Dry skin | *Actinobacteria*, *Firmicutes*, *Proteobacteria*, and *Bacteroidetes* |
| | Moist skin | *Staphylococcus* and *Corynebacterium* |
| | Seborrhoeic skin | *Propionibacterium* |

The number of bacteria that colonise the human body is estimated at 10 times the number of human cells. These microbes, in addition to colonising, contain functional genes responsible for synthesising numerous metabolites that can influence the health of the host. It is estimated that human skin is inhabited by approximately 1 million bacteria per $cm^2$, and by smaller numbers of fungi and viruses.

It is crucial to be familiar with the normal microbiota of our patients in order to understand the imbalances that occur in the majority of skin disorders. This knowledge will also help us develop future strategies to control secondary cutaneous infections and ultimately decrease our reliance on antimicrobial agents. When used continuously and excessively, antimicrobial agents contribute to the appearance of multiresistant organisms, which complicate the resolution of secondary factors present in many skin disorders.

> Studies of the cutaneous microbiome have proliferated in the last decade.

The microbiome is unique and exhibits significant differences in bacterial species associated with age, sex, hygiene, lifestyle, and even the environment.

## Bacterial skin infections

Cutaneous bacteria reside in the superficial epidermis and the infundibulum of the hair follicles, where sweat and sebum provide nutrients. The normal biota consists of a mixture of bacteria that live in symbiosis. The makeup of the biota can change depending on the status of the skin (i.e. in response to factors such as heat, pH, salinity, humidity, and albumin and fatty acid levels).

In cats, and to a greater extent in dogs, bacterial skin infections are one of the most frequent causes of complications in different skin disorders. These infections are usually considered secondary complications. They can affect different strata of the skin and can vary in severity.

> **Most skin infections in dogs have an underlying cause, which can be inflammatory, due to a keratinisation disorder, or secondary, due to cutaneous parasitosis.**

When there is clinical evidence of a bacterial infection, the veterinary surgeon should always consider the primary factor that triggered it, and use diagnostic tools to find and correct this primary cause in order to prevent the development of bacterial complications.

## Resident or transient bacteria

Bacteria isolated from normal skin are known as normal inhabitants, and can be classified as transient or resident based on their ability to multiply in the habitat in question.

### Resident bacteria

Resident bacteria (Table 2) have the ability to multiply on normal skin. Some studies have enabled differentiation of resident bacteria from those present due to repeated contamination of the skin.

### Transient bacteria

Transient bacteria can be isolated from the skin, but are of no clinical significance unless they become invasive and contribute to a pathological process, since they do not normally multiply on the skin of most animals. Transient bacteria found in dogs include *Escherichia coli*, *Proteus mirabilis*, *Corynebacterium* spp., *Bacillus* spp., *Pseudomonas* spp., and coagulase-positive staphylococci.

**Table 2.** Resident bacteria in different areas of the skin.

<table>
<tr><th colspan="2">Anatomical area</th><th>Resident bacteria</th></tr>
<tr><td colspan="2">Skin surface</td><td>Micrococcus spp., coagulase-negative staphylococcus (especially Staphylococcus epidermidis and Staphylococcus xylosus), α-haemolytic streptococcus, Clostridium spp., Propionibacterium acnes, Acinetobacter spp., and several gram-negative aerobes.</td></tr>
<tr><td rowspan="2">Hair</td><td>Hair shafts</td><td>Micrococcus spp., gram-negative aerobes, Bacillus spp., and Staphylococcus pseudintermedius.</td></tr>
<tr><td>Hair follicle</td><td>Micrococcus spp., P. acnes, streptococci, Bacillus spp., and S. pseudintermedius.</td></tr>
</table>

### Canine atopic dermatitis and dysbiosis

Canine atopic dermatitis is a chronic, pruritic inflammatory disease with a genetic component, and is characterised by the generation of specific IgE against different environmental or food allergens, to which the patient becomes sensitised. This generates a cutaneous and pruriginous inflammatory process that gives rise to secondary infections caused by commensal bacteria and/or yeast.

In some cases, dogs can become sensitised to *Staphylococcus pseudintermedius* or *Malassezia pachydermatis*, two of the main organisms that cause secondary infections in patients with atopic dermatitis. This results in a worsening of the clinical signs in the presence of these secondary agents, generating a greater inflammatory and pruritic response in patients with these infections. The skin lesions are exacerbated by the presence of these bacteria, giving rise to papules, pustules, or crusts.

## Diagnosis of bacterial skin infections

### Skin cytology

Cytology is one of the most important tools in dermatological diagnosis. It provides a large amount of information and is the most commonly used test in dermatological practice.

Skin cytology is defined as the microscopic evaluation of cells and organisms located on the skin surface. In addition to providing a wealth of information, it is much less expensive than many other tests (e.g. biopsy, bacterial culture, fungal culture).

It constitutes a valuable source of information for the clinic, owing to its low cost, its diagnostic value, and the possibility of repeat analyses, which enable monitoring of the process and modification of treatment based on the cytological findings.

Using basic cytology, the clinician will be able to identify microorganisms present in skin samples and to therefore differentiate between bacteria and yeast.

## Collection of samples

Different materials are used to collect samples for skin cytology:

- Swabs
- Slides
- Spatula
- Scalpel blade
- 26-gauge or 22-gauge needle
- Transparent tape

**It is important to select the appropriate technique to collect the sample, depending on the type of lesion or anatomical location.**

## Direct impression with a slide

Direct impression with a slide is this author's preferred technique. It is fast and practical, and provides valuable information without resulting in excessive contamination with particles or residues.

It is performed by applying light to moderate pressure on the lesion, which may be located beneath a crust (Fig. 1). Other lesion types for which this technique can be used are epidermal collarettes (Fig. 2) and exudative, ulcerative, pustular (Fig. 3), and papular (Fig. 4) lesions. However, direct impression is unsuitable for collecting samples from the interdigital spaces, since these areas are difficult to access with a slide. Similarly, this technique is not recommended for dry exfoliative lesions, since these do not allow adhesion of cytological material to the slide. However, it can be used to acquire samples from some exfoliative lesions (Fig. 5).

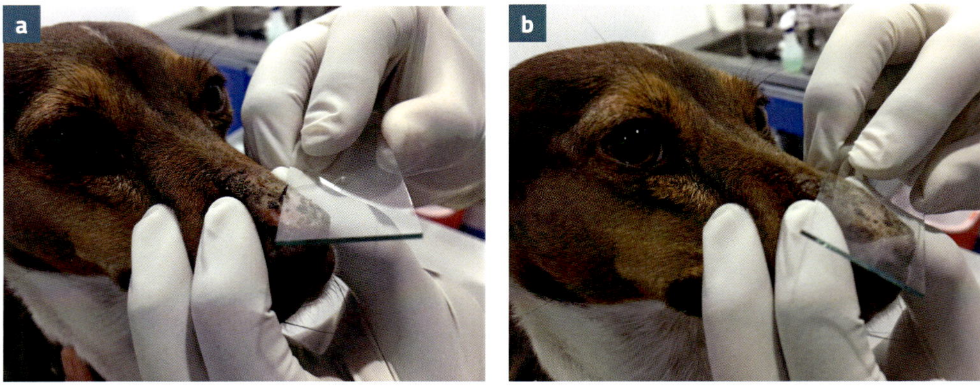

Figure 1. Direct impression of a crusted lesion located on the nasal bridge. (a) The slide can be used to lift the crust from the lesion. (b) An impression smear of the lesion under the crust is made with the slide.

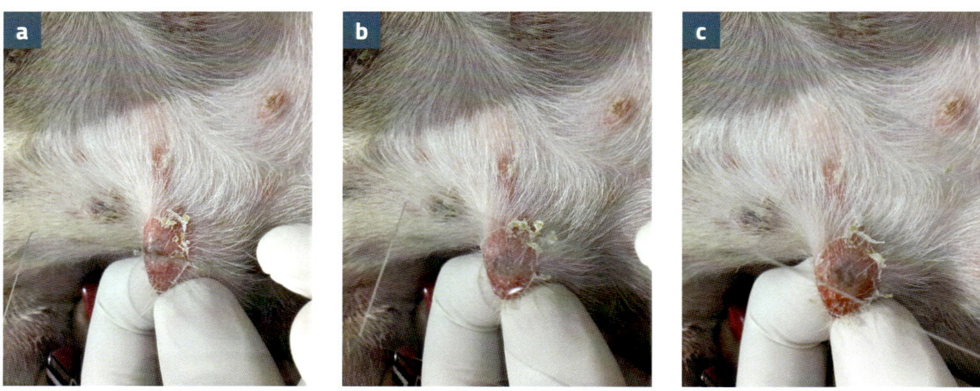

Figure 2. Direct impression of an epidermal collarette. (a) (b) The edge of the slide is used to lift the edge of the lesion. (c) A smear of the lesion is made by applying moderate pressure with the slide against the edge of the epidermal collarette.

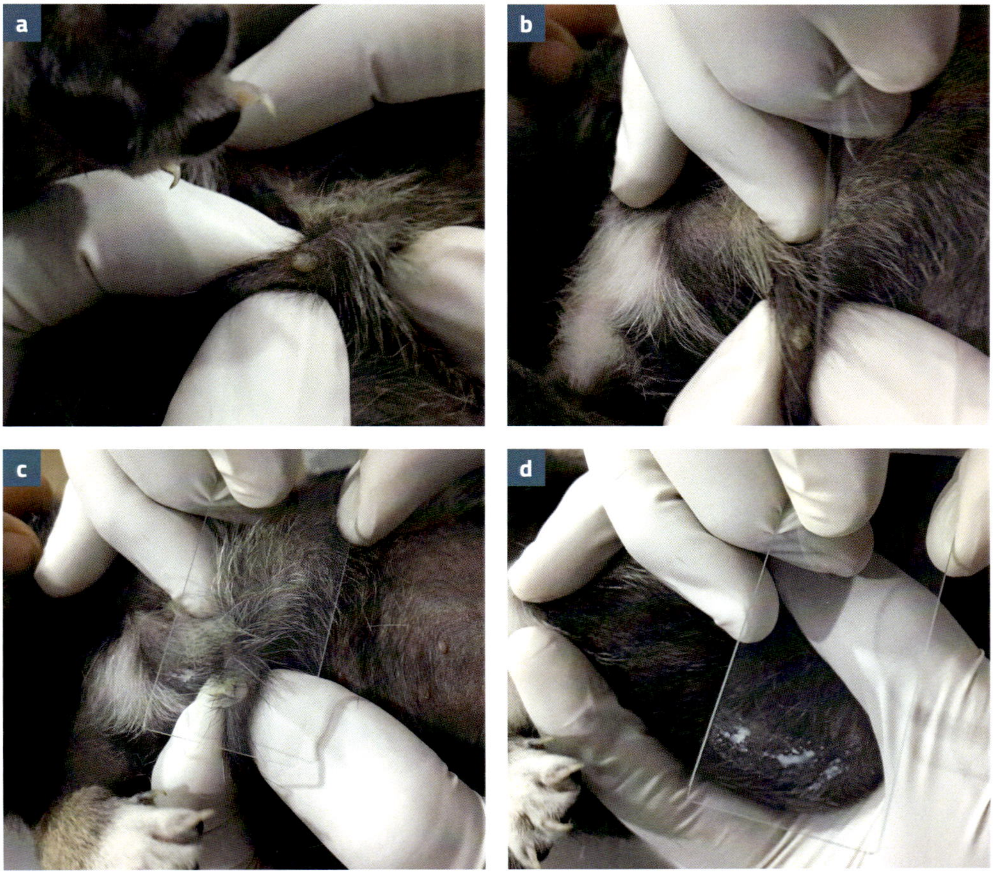


Figure 3. Direct impression of a pustular lesion. (a) Appearance of the lesion. (b) The pustule is opened with the edge of the slide. (c, d) At the same time, the slide is pressed and moved across the lesion to collect material.

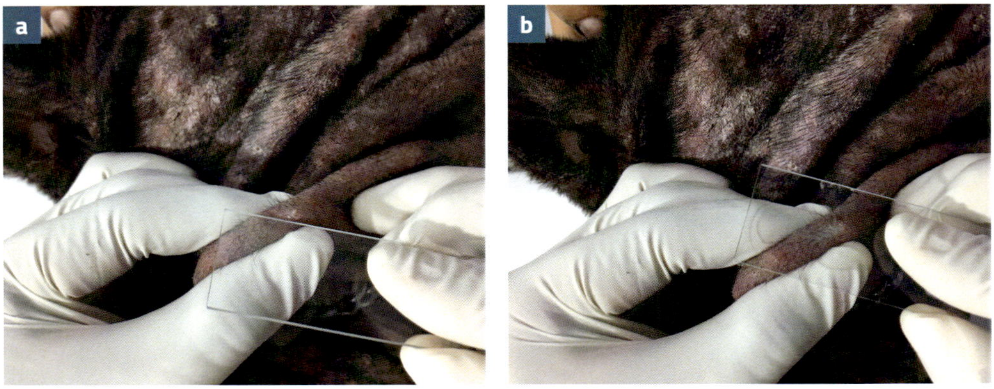


Figure 4. Direct impression of a papular lesion. (a) The slide is used to obtain the impression smear. (b) At the same time, the slide is moved across the lesion.

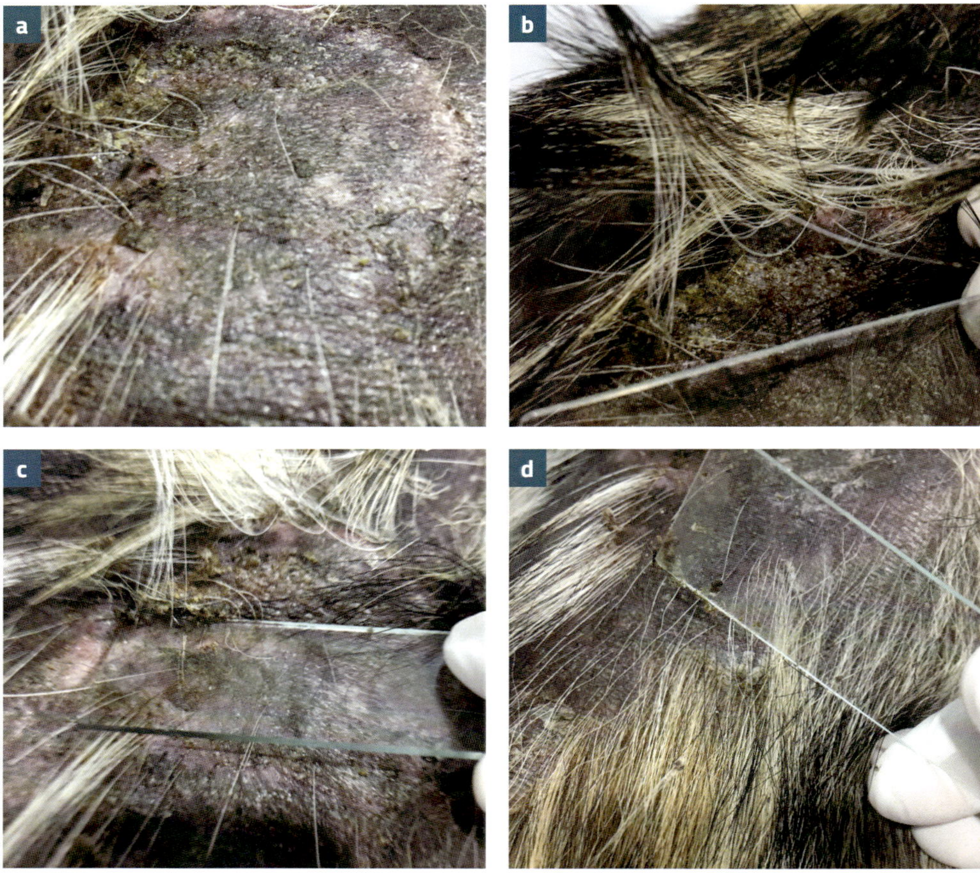


**Figure 5.** Direct impression of an exfoliative lesion. (a) Appearance of the lesion. (b) The edge of the slide is used to scrape the lesion. (c, d) While scraping, light-to-moderate pressure is applied to obtain a smear of the area in contact with the slide.

## Adhesive tape cytology

Transparent or acetate tape impression is used for a variety of applications in the field of veterinary dermatology. This technique is most commonly used as a complementary technique together with skin scraping and the collection of material for cytological evaluation.

Tape strip cytology is a very economical, easy to perform, and diagnostically valuable technique. The only material required is transparent acetate tape, like that used in offices.

Acetate tape is particularly useful to collect material for cytological evaluation from dry lesions and hard-to-reach areas in which direct impression is not possible. These areas include the nail bed, interdigital spaces (Figs. 6 and 7), the periocular area, and skinfolds. Once the sample is taken, the tape strip is stuck to one end of a slide, which serves as a handle during the subsequent staining process (Figs. 7 and 14).

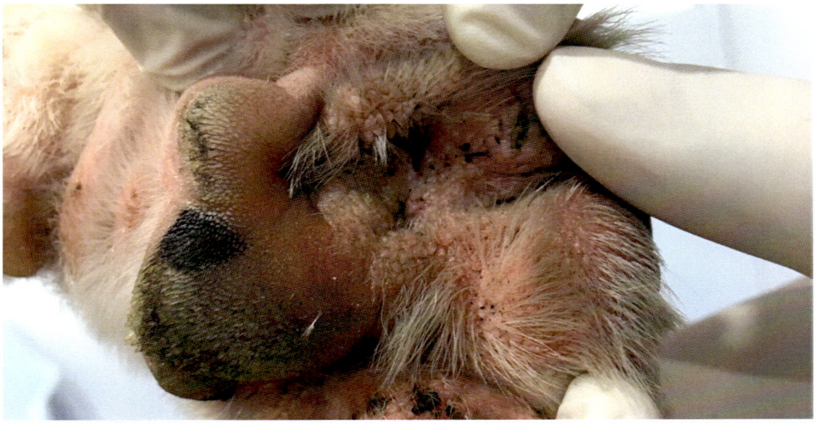

**Figure 6.** Erythema and inflammation between the footpads of an English Bulldog with canine atopic dermatitis.

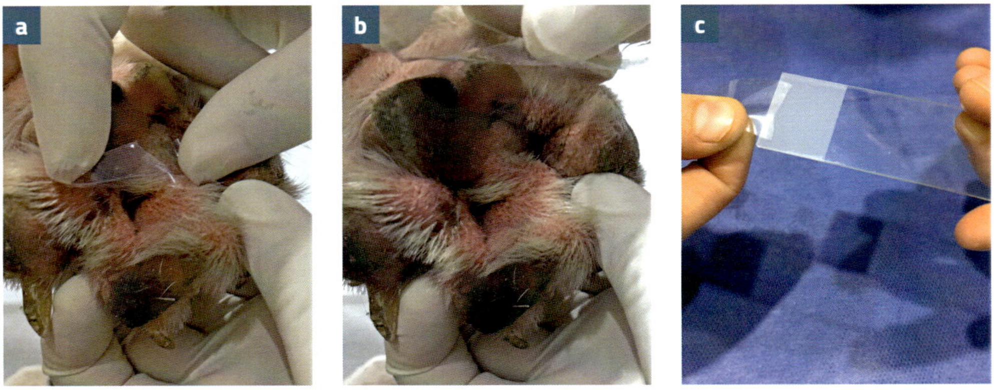

**Figure 7.** Collection of material for cytological evaluation using transparent tape. (a) The tape is placed on the affected area and pressure exerted on the site to be sampled. (b) The tape is then peeled off and (c) attached to one end of the slide, which serves as a handle during the staining process.

## Tzanck technique

This collection technique consists of puncturing a pustular, vesicular, or bullous lesion with a needle and transferring the collected material on a slide (Fig. 8).

The advantage of this technique over direct impression is that there is no significant risk of bacterial contamination, since care is taken to avoid contact with the skin surrounding the lesion.

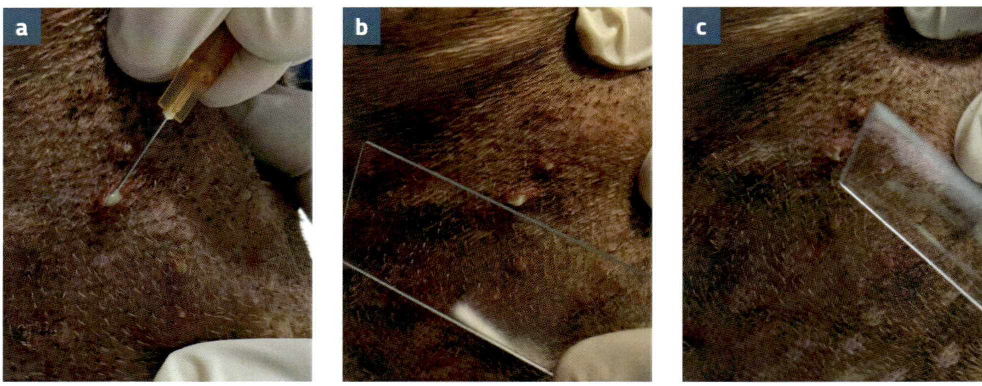

**Figure 8.** Sampling of a pustular lesion using the Tzanck technique. (a) The pustule is punctured with a 26-gauge needle. (b) The material is collected using a slide or the needle itself, avoiding contact with the skin. (c) The collected material is spread on the slide.

## Nail bed cytology

The nail bed is an area that is overlooked by some clinicians. However, in allergic patients (Fig. 9) yeast and bacterial infections can develop in this area, resulting in pruritus.

> If signs of pruritus, inflammation, or discolouration are observed in the nail bed or at the base of the nail, cytology should be performed.

Samples for nail bed cytology can be collected using the edge of a slide (Fig. 10), although this technique can often cause damage in the area. Alternatives include a toothpick, as mentioned in a recent study (Rosenkrantz, 2016), a metal spatula (Fig. 11), or even transparent tape (Fig. 12).

If a toothpick or spatula is used, the collected material is then spread on a slide.

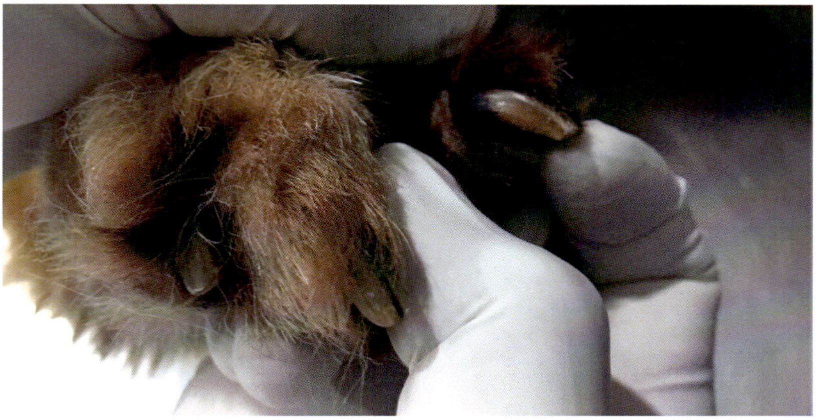

Figure 9. Nail bed displaying inflammation and discolouration at the base of the nail.

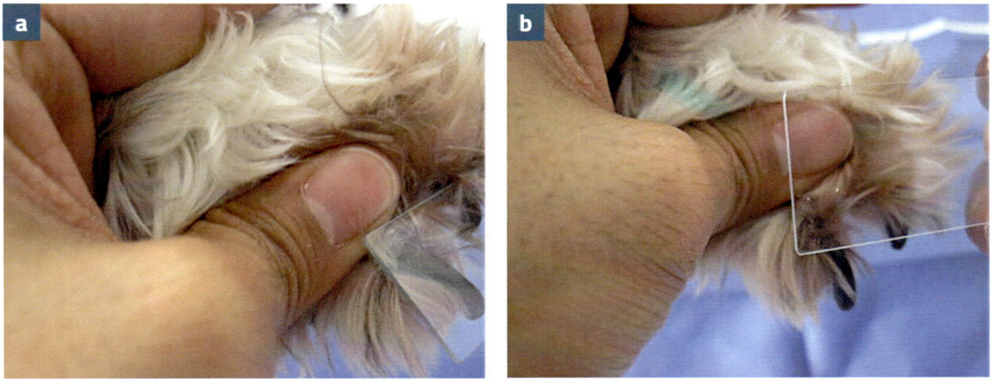

Figure 10. Sampling of the nail bed using a slide. (a) The material is collected by pressing a slide against the area of interest. (b) The collected material remains adhered to the slide.

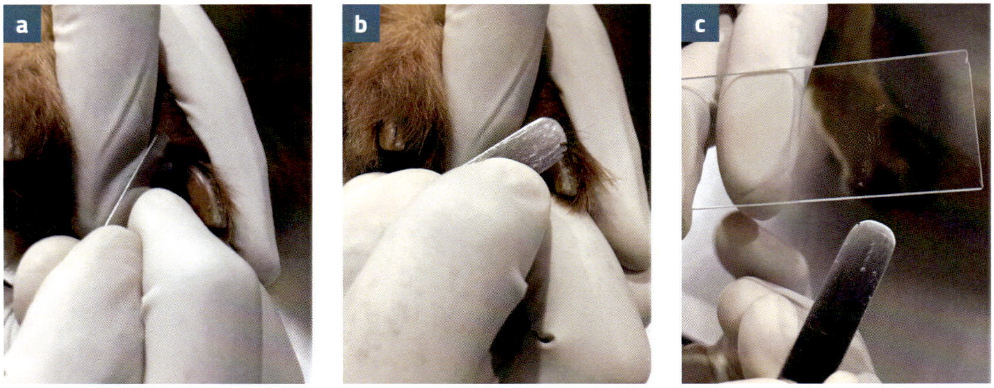

Figure 11. Sample collection from the nail bed and base of the nail with a metal spatula. (a) A spatula is used to perform a light scraping. (b) The material is collected. (c) The material is spread on a slide.

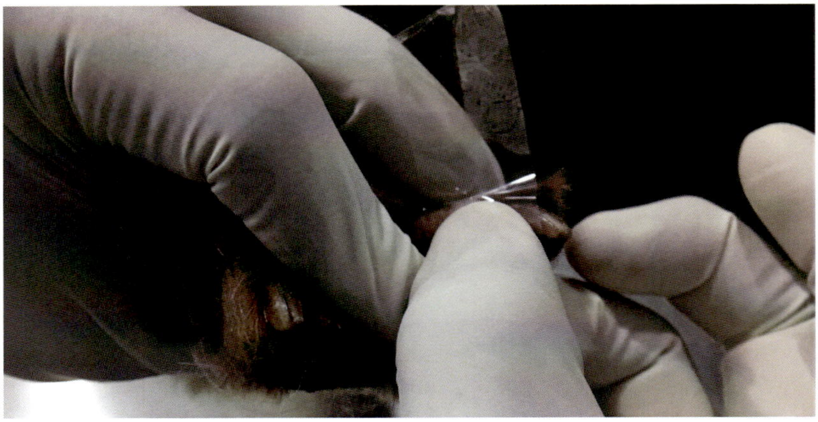

**Figure 12.** To collect samples from the nail bed with transparent tape, the tape is stuck to the area of interest and then detached.

## Staining

Once the sample has been collected for cytology, it is then stained. The most commonly used staining methods in dermatology are Diff-Quik or Hemacolor rapid staining (Figs. 13 and 14) and new methylene blue. Diff-Quik is a Romanowsky-type stain that provides less nuclear detail than supravital stains, but allows good cytoplasmic differentiation and visualisation of cytoplasmic structures and microorganisms. Since most of the diseases to be evaluated will be nonneoplastic, it is the method of choice.

Gram staining can be used to evaluate bacteria, especially in otic samples, but provides no added value and is less practical than Diff-Quik.

Staining using the Diff-Quik method requires three distinct solutions: a fixative solution (1), a red solution (2), and a purple solution (3). The sample is introduced for 5 seconds 3 times in each solution following the sequence 1, 2, and 3, without returning to the previous solution. However, this author prefers to submerge the sample for 15–20 seconds in each solution. Once the sample is stained, it is rinsed with distilled water or preferably with running tap water, and is left to dry. Once dry, the sample can be observed under the microscope. Samples can be fixed with resin and coverslipped in order to preserve them for future study or to add them to a collection.

**Diff-Quik or rapid Hemacolor staining**

- In samples taken from the ear or in cases in which fatty material is obtained it is necessary to fix the sample before staining.
- If the objective is solely to identify microorganisms (yeast, bacteria), the first two solutions (1 and 2) can be omitted and only the blue solution (3) used. However, it is advisable to complete all three steps in order to perform a complete cytological evaluation.

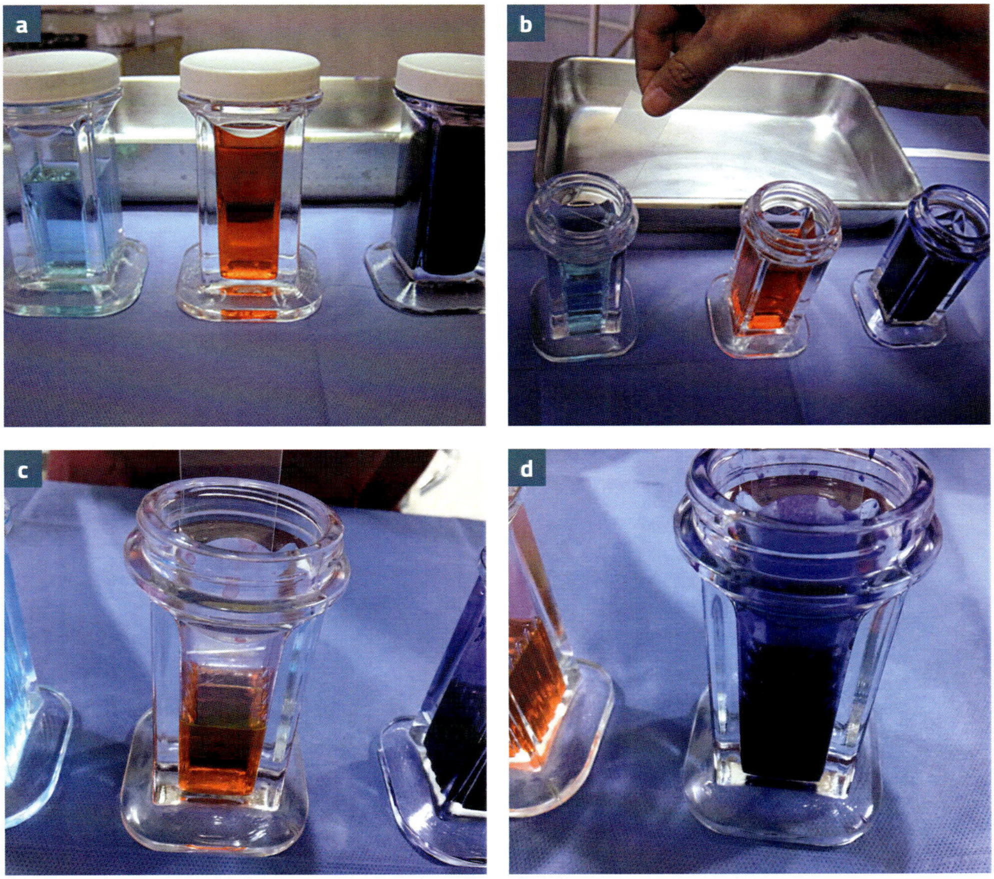


**Figure 13.** Diff-Quik or Hemacolor rapid staining. (a) Fixative solution, red solution, and purple solution. (b) The slide bearing the sample is immersed in the fixative solution. (c) The excess fixative solution is drained from the slide, which is then immersed in the red solution. (d) Next, the slide is immersed in the purple solution. Finally, the sample is cleared and dried for microscopic observation.

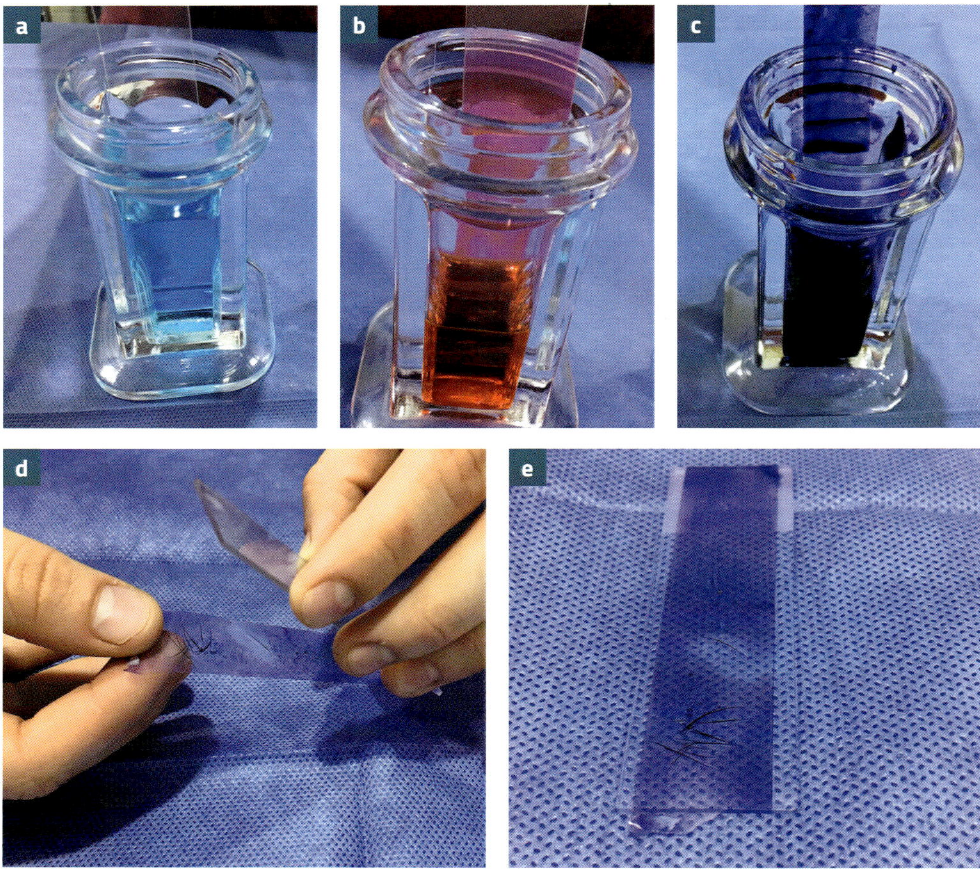


**Figure 14.** Staining of a cytology sample acquired using transparent tape and mounting for evaluation under the microscope. (a–c) The tape attached to the slide is stained using the Diff-Quik method. (d, e) The stained tape is placed on the slide, with the cytological material facing the slide. Next, the slide is observed under the microscope.

## Microscopic observation

One of the most expensive pieces of equipment required for skin cytology, and for other diagnostic tests in dermatology, is the microscope. Although costs can vary, a microscope represents an important long-term investment for the clinician, and if well used provides considerable value even in the short term.

Ideally, a microscope should be binocular. When selecting a microscope the optics, the quality of the materials, and even the customer service offered by the manufacturer should be taken into account.

When evaluating cytological samples the condenser of the microscope should be adjusted to allow entry of a larger beam of light (Fig. 15). Initially, samples are observed using the dry 4× objective to evaluate the most populated fields on the slide. Next, the 10× or 40× objective can be used. These objectives do not allow easy visualisation of microorganisms or examination of nuclear detail, but provide the trained clinician with information on cell types, and allow evaluation of cells on the periphery.

Most cytology samples are evaluated using the 100× objective (Fig. 16), which requires the use of immersion oil. To do this, it is necessary to partially switch objectives and deposit a drop of immersion oil on the slide. Next, the 100× objective is placed in the viewing position and then focused by adjusting the objective as required.

There are three types of immersion oils: A, B, and NVH. Each differs in viscosity: type A is the least viscous and type NVH is the most viscous. Type B is the most commonly used, although type A is preferable as it is the easiest to clean.

Care should be taken when focusing the 100× objective; lowering the objective too far can result in damage to the slide and/or lens. The 40× objective should not be used over areas to which immersion oil has been applied in order to prevent soiling of the lens, which is positioned very close to the slide.

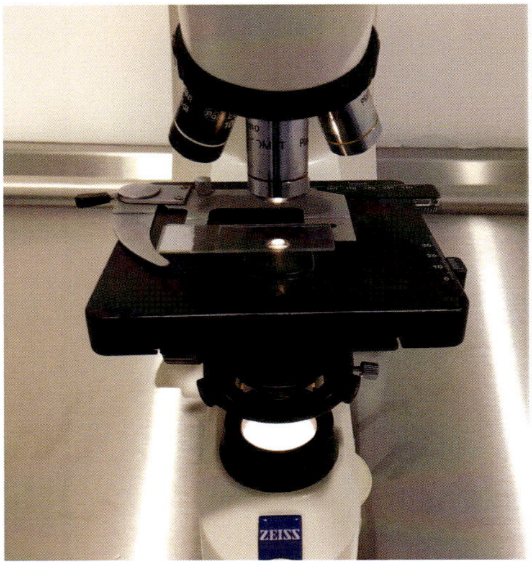


**Figure 15.** In contrast to skin scrapings or trichograms, cytological samples should be observed under the microscope with the condenser open. This allows for greater passage of light.

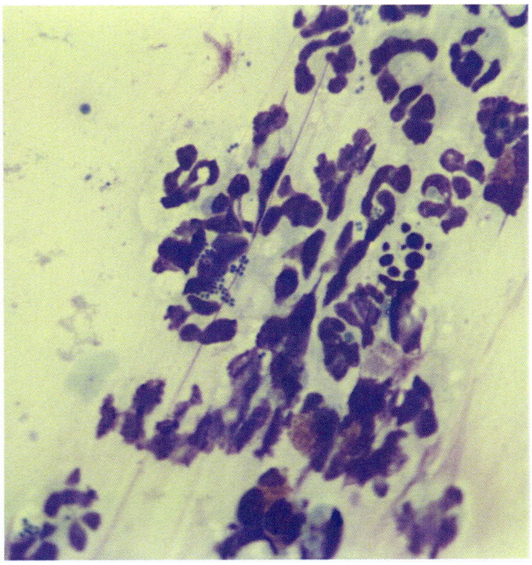

**Figure 16.** Microscopic observation with a 100× objective of a sample collected with acetate tape. Abundant coccoid bacteria that have been phagocytosed by neutrophils are observed.

## SUMMARY

- Bacterial infections usually have an underlying cause that should be identified and controlled.
- Cytology helps the veterinary surgeon make better decisions regarding the treatment of bacterial infections.
- The most appropriate sampling technique should be selected for each type of lesion.
- It is preferable to use rapid stains that allow good visualisation of the sample.

02

# SUPERFICIAL BACTERIAL INFECTIONS

A soon as one understands the importance of the microbiota and its fundamental role in the cutaneous ecosystem, as well as the techniques necessary to collect samples for the diagnosis of bacterial skin infections, the next step is to understand how these infections are classified according to depth. This chapter will focus on surface and superficial pyoderma.

Surface pyoderma includes pyotraumatic and intertrigo dermatitis, although pyotraumatic dermatitis can be considered a form of deep pyoderma depending on its severity.

Superficial pyoderma, as the term suggests, refers to infections that affect the epidermis and the follicular epithelium. These infections can be classified as impetigo, mucocutaneous pyoderma, or superficial bacterial folliculitis.

## Pyotraumatic dermatitis

Pyotraumatic dermatitis (also known as hot spot) often has an acute onset and is typically the result of self-induced trauma in response to pain or itching that causes the patient to scratch or lick a specific area.

### Skin lesions

The characteristic lesion is red, exudative, and moist, and is usually associated with a central protein clot and surrounded by an erythematous halo (Fig. 1). Hair is absent from the affected area, but well-defined margins surrounded by normal skin are visible. The lesion is painful and progresses rapidly if left untreated. The hair in the surrounding area should be clipped to facilitate evaluation and the collection of samples for cytology (Figs. 2 and 3).

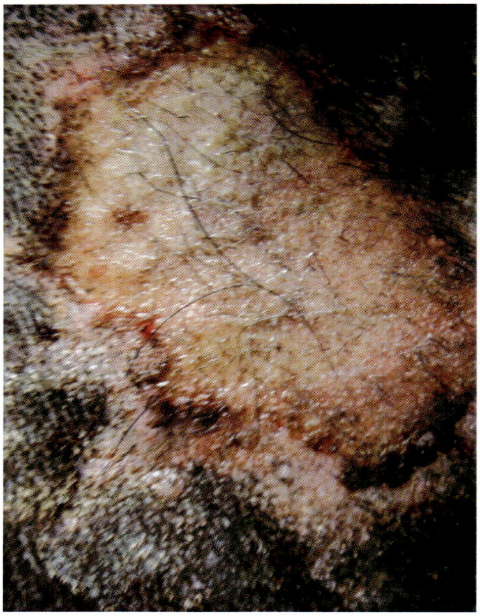

**Figure 1.** Superficial pyotraumatic dermatitis (hot spot) in which the well-delimited borders and the yellow crust are evident.

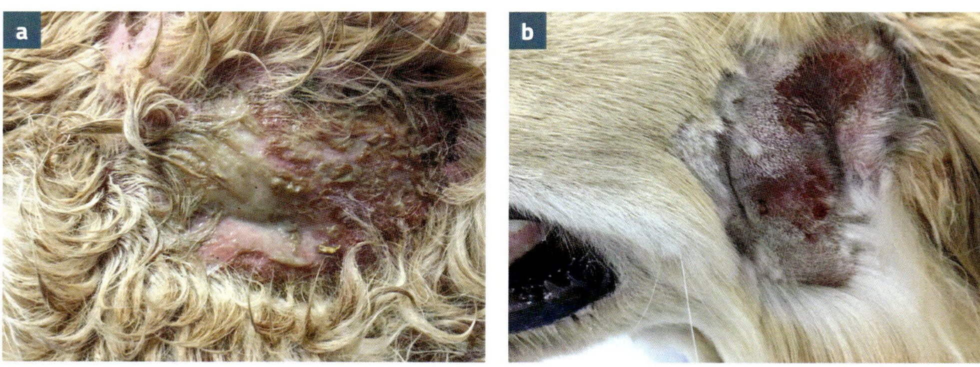


**Figure 2.** Pyotraumatic dermatitis. (a) Lesion (before clipping) with an evident protein clot. Note the hair adhering to the lesion surface. (b) Lesion (after clipping) with no satellite papules.

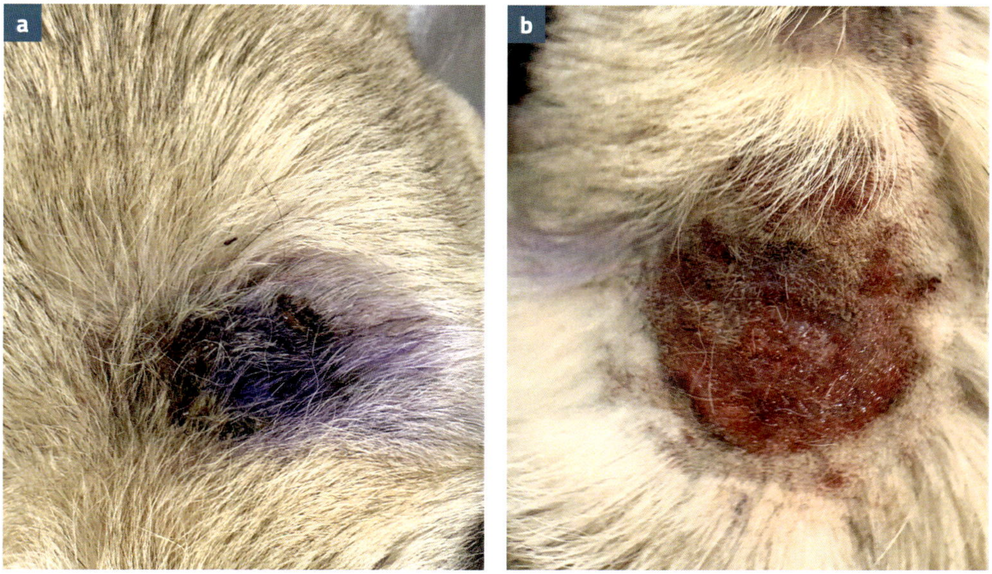


**Figure 3.** Pyotraumatic dermatitis. (a) Appearance of the lesion before clipping. (b) Lesion after clipping. Note the satellite papules around the central lesion.

## Diagnostic findings

Diagnosis is based on the patient's clinical history, the physical appearance of the lesion, its date of appearance, and any associated primary cause.

Cytology can reveal colonisation of the skin surface by bacteria, in the absence of the characteristic features of bacterial infection. Infection may be observed in cases of deeper lesions that progress to pyotraumatic folliculitis or furunculosis. Biopsy of chronic lesions may be necessary to differentiate between superficial and deep pyotraumatic dermatitis.

> Infection should be suspected if papules are observed around the central lesion (satellite papules) or if the lesion thickens to form a plaque.

## Therapeutic management

Therapeutic management includes clipping the surrounding hair and cleaning the lesion with antibacterial agents. For deeper lesions, systemic antibiotic therapy, in some cases combined with oral or topical corticosteroids, may be required.

## Intertrigo

Intertrigo or skinfold dermatitis usually occurs in poorly ventilated areas and is the result of irritation caused by friction between two skin surfaces. The presence of moisture, sebum, glandular secretions, or excretions such as tears, saliva, or urine gives rise to an environment conducive to tissue maceration and overgrowth of bacteria or yeast of the genus *Malassezia*.

**Intertrigo usually affects obese animals and breeds with characteristic skinfolds.**

### Skin lesions

Inflammation, marked erythema, and even brownish or yellowish discharge may be observed within the skinfolds (Figs. 4 and 5). This condition is usually accompanied by a foul smell and pain on palpation.

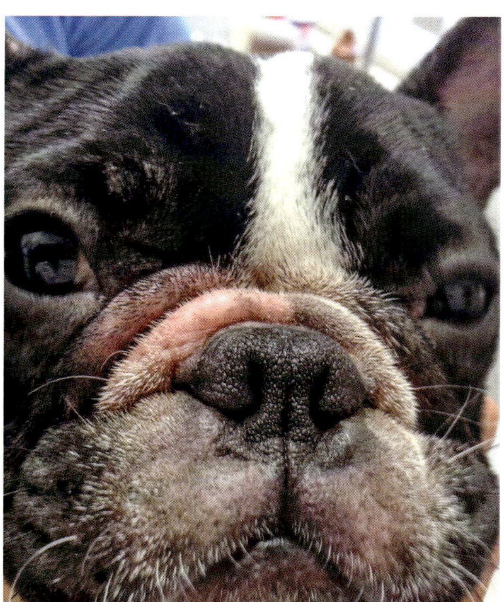

**Figure 4.** Facial intertrigo in a French Bulldog with atopic dermatitis.

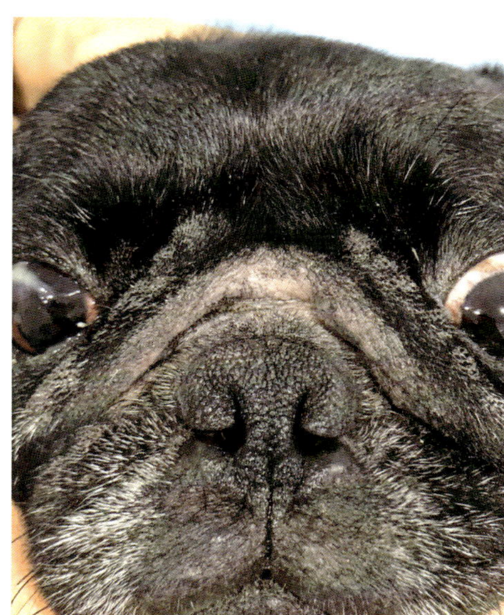

**Figure 5.** Facial intertrigo in a Pug.

### Diagnostic findings

Cytology may reveal bacterial or yeast overgrowth with few or no inflammatory cells. Phagocytosis is usually not observed.

### Therapeutic management

The affected area should be cleaned with antibacterial or antifungal products combined with antiseptic agents if *Malassezia* is present. Topical or oral corticosteroids administered at anti-inflammatory doses may also be required.

If the skinfolds cannot be eliminated by surgery or treatment of obesity, areas predisposed to intertrigo should be periodically cleaned.

## Impetigo

Impetigo is characterised by the presence of nonfollicular subcorneal pustules that affect areas with little hair.

In most cases there is no apparent cause, although impetigo more often affects puppies with parasitic or viral diseases, poor nutrition, or poor hygiene.

> Puppies are affected at young ages, usually before or during the onset of sexual maturity.

In cases in which adult or senior dogs are affected bullous impetigo should be considered. This can be caused by bacteria of the genus *Pseudomonas* or by *Escherichia coli*, and can be associated with hypercortisolism, diabetes mellitus, hypothyroidism, and other debilitating diseases. In these patients it is advisable to carry out a complete health assessment.

### Skin lesions

The most common impetigo lesions are pustules with no hair follicle involvement. These types of lesions can be the primary lesion, although owing to its fragility it is common to observe epidermal collarettes with a yellowish crust in areas with little hair (usually the abdominal area), in some cases with mild central hyperpigmentation (Fig. 6).

These pustules are neither pruritic nor painful, although itching may be caused by the presence of some follicular pustules. In kittens, lesions are usually found on the back of the neck, the head, or the interscapular area.

It is important to examine the content of the pustules under a microscope, without staining. The condenser of the microscope should be adjusted to reduce the entry of light and ensure greater contrast in order to detect the possible presence of demodicosis, especially in cases of widespread pustular lesions with a predominance of follicular pustules. One report described a case of pustular demodicosis in a 2-week old litter of Pug puppies.

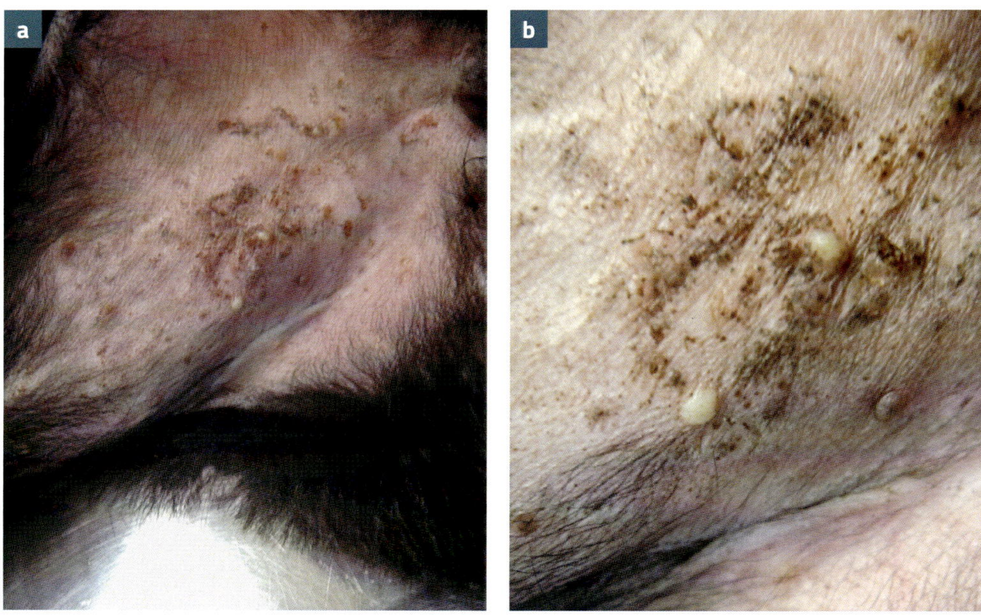


**Figure 6.** Abdominal impetigo in a puppy. (a) Subcorneal pustules and hyperpigmented lesions produced by the rupture of the former. (b) Magnified image of the lesions. The subcorneal pustules can cover several follicles.

## Diagnostic findings

Cytology may reveal neutrophilic inflammation with the presence of bacteria (cocci or bacilli). Histology shows subcorneal nonfollicular pustules with or without the presence of bacteria.

In bullous impetigo, histology reveals discrete subcorneal or intragranular pustules composed mainly of neutrophils and in some cases affecting several follicles, and mild separation of keratinocytes (acantholysis). The acantholysis can be deep in some cases.

The characteristics, especially the acantholysis, are very similar to those of pemphigus foliaceus. Caution is thus advised to avoid a misdiagnosis of autoimmune disease.

### Therapeutic management

In some cases impetigo can spontaneously regress. However, treatment can accelerate the recovery process or help control lesion proliferation in cases in which regression does not occur. Usually, topical treatment is indicated.

When lesions are grouped (which is rare), gels, creams, or ointments containing mupirocin, fusidic acid, or chlorhexidine can be used. However, because the affected areas tend to be extensive, the most practical treatments are antibacterial shampoos (chlorhexidine, ethyl lactate, or benzoyl peroxide).

Because the skin of puppies is easily irritated, caution is required when using products such as benzoyl peroxide. This author prefers 3 % or 4 % chlorhexidine, preferably in products that also contain ceramides.

The affected area should be washed every day or every other day for 1 to 2 weeks. If the lesion does not resolve, systemic antibiotics can be administered, following the guidelines provided in Chapter 8.

## Mucocutaneous pyoderma

Mucocutaneous pyoderma is a frequently recurrent skin condition, the aetiology of which remains unclear. It affects the lips, perioral skin, nasal plane, and nostrils (Figs. 7–12). Other areas that may also be affected include the eyelids (Fig. 13), vulva, foreskin, and anus.

**The German Shepherd and its crosses are predisposed to this skin condition.**

## Skin lesions

The variable clinical presentation of mucocutaneous pyoderma can include erythema and inflammation that progresses to crusts, fissures, erosion, ulceration, and localised depigmentation.

This skin condition can be easily confused with labial intertrigo, although in the latter, which more commonly affects Spaniels, ulcerative lesions are absent. In some cases, mucocutaneous pyoderma may be associated with an underlying disease (e.g. atopic dermatitis).

## Diagnostic findings

Diagnosis is confirmed based on clinical, cytological, and histological findings.

Cytology may reveal predominantly neutrophilic inflammation, with or without the presence of macrophages, and abundant bacteria, which can include buccal bacteria such as bacilli or even *Simonsiella* spp. (Fig. 14).

Histology shows epidermal hyperplasia with pustules and superficial crusts. Dense, mainly plasmacytic lichenoid dermatitis, prominent neutrophils, and even pigmentary incontinence are observed in the dermis.

## Therapeutic management

Mucocutaneous pyoderma responds to topical or systemic antibacterial treatment. However, the response is often slow and relapse is not uncommon.

In the case of topical treatment, hair in the periphery of the affected area should be clipped to facilitate administration. Benzoyl peroxide, chlorhexidine, or other antibacterial agents can be used. After cleaning the lesions, antibacterial mupirocin ointment or cream can be applied. Treatment should be administered for at least 14 days.

In severe cases of mucocutaneous pyoderma, systemic antibiotic treatment for 3 to 4 weeks may be necessary.

Mucocutaneous pyoderma affecting the nasal plane can resemble discoid lupus erythematosus both clinically and histologically. Therefore, in cases in which these conditions are clinically suspected, a failure to respond to antibiotic therapy should be verified before instituting immunosuppressive treatment.

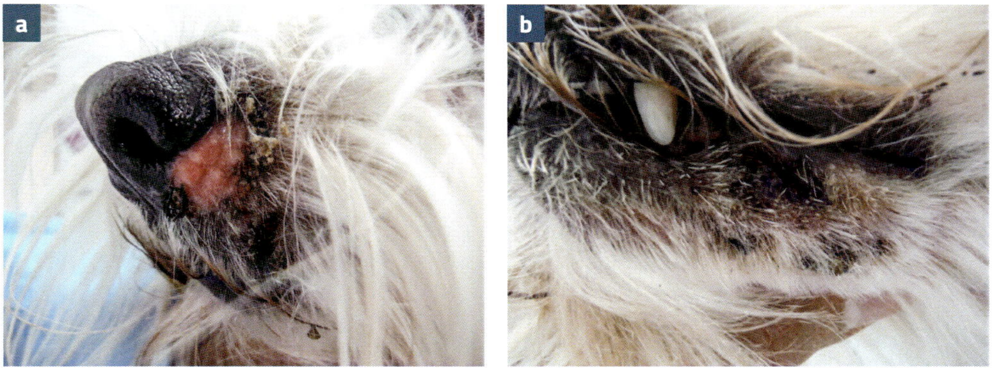

Figure 7. Mucocutaneous pyoderma in a patient with presumptive diagnosis of autoimmune dermatosis. (a) Involvement of the nasal area and presence of crusted lesions. (b) Inflammation and crusted lesions in the perilabial area. The patient exhibited pain on palpation of the affected areas.

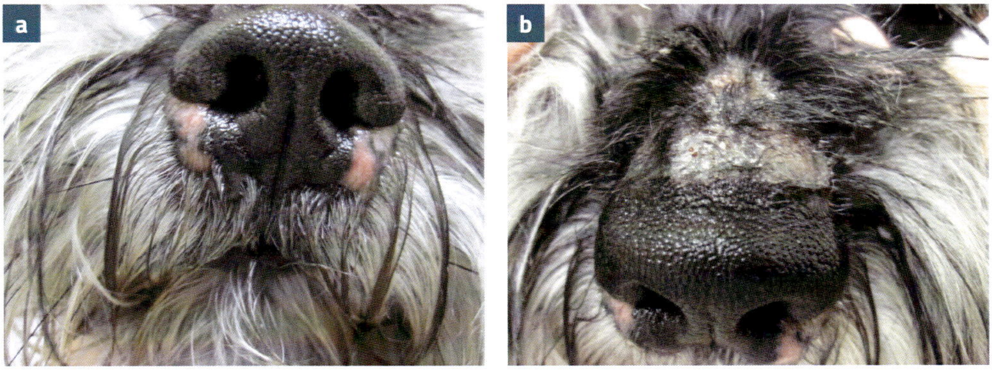

Figure 8. Mucocutaneous pyoderma with nasal involvement. (a) Areas of depigmentation that can be mistaken for signs of autoimmune dermatosis. (b) Crusted and inflammatory lesions on the nasal plane.

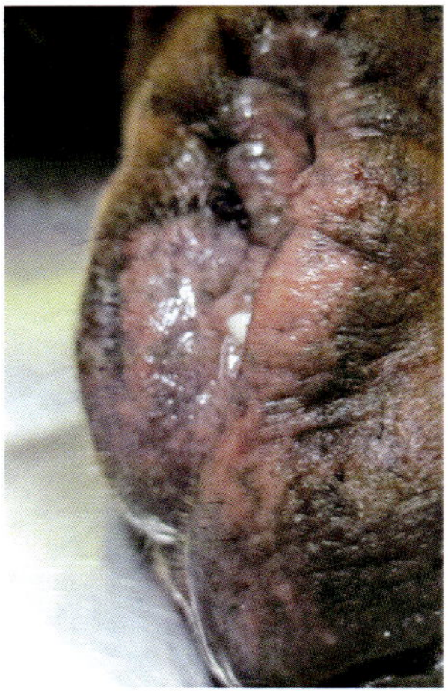

Figure 9. Perilabial area of a Dachshund with mucocutaneous pyoderma.

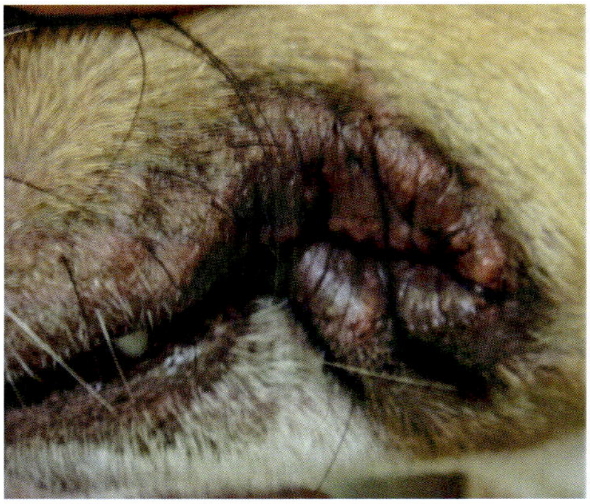

Figure 10. Perilabial mucocutaneous pyoderma with ulceration and skinfold lesions.

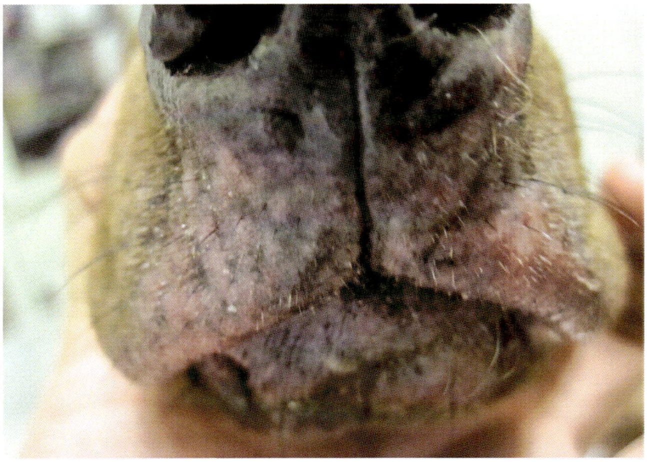

**Figure 11.** Mucocutaneous pyoderma affecting the chin area.

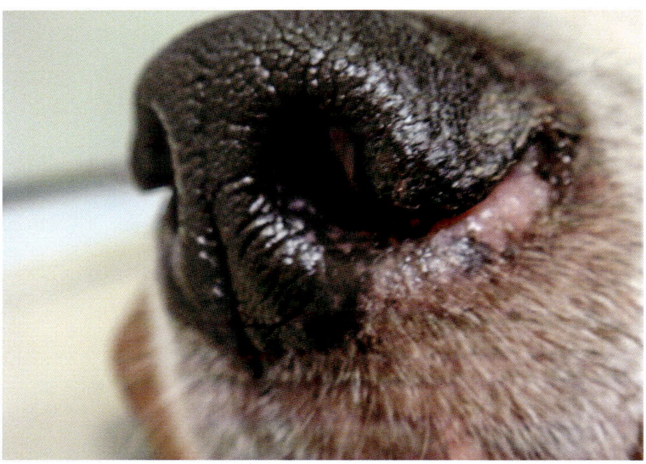

**Figure 12.** Nasal mucocutaneous pyoderma with depigmentation lesions around the nasal margins.

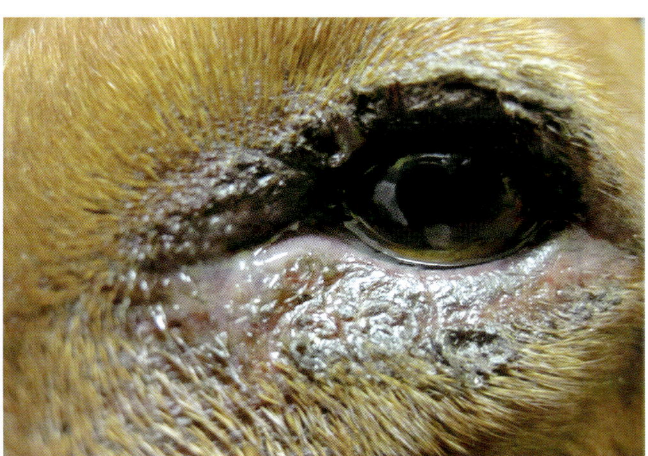

**Figure 13.** Periocular mucocutaneous pyoderma.

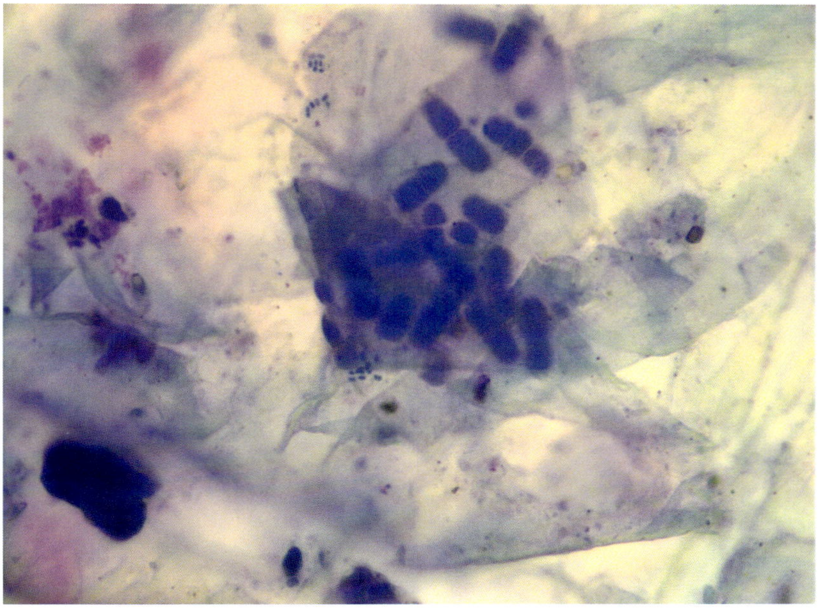

Figure 14. Cytology reveals the presence of *Simonsiella* spp. in a patient with superficial pyoderma. These organisms are usually part of the oral microbiota and appear as a result of secondary contamination in areas that are frequent licked.

## Superficial bacterial folliculitis

Superficial bacterial folliculitis is the most common form of pyoderma in dogs, and the main reason for the use of antibiotics in small animal practice. When dealing with this condition, it is therefore important to develop a habit of rational use of antibiotics in daily practice. This issue is dealt with thoroughly in the final chapter of this book.

In most cases, superficial bacterial folliculitis is caused by *Staphylococcus pseudintermedius*, although other *Staphylococcus* species can also be involved. These microorganisms can be introduced into the skin through trauma, scratching, or injury, or by infection as a consequence of poor hygiene, seborrhoea, parasitic infestation (especially demodicosis), hormonal factors, local irritants, or allergies. The three most common causes of folliculitis are bacteria, dermatophytes, and parasites (*Demodex*).

**Superficial bacterial folliculitis can progress to deep folliculitis, furunculosis, and even cellulitis.**

For reasons that remain unclear, pruritus may or may not be present. A greater pruritic component is indicative of a potential underlying allergic cause.

## Skin lesions

There is no characteristic lesion distribution pattern or typical clinical presentation. Because the infection is secondary, the area affected will vary depending on the underlying cause.

In cases of trauma or laceration, lesions tend to appear in the area of the injury. When the underlying causes are systemic, lesions tend to predominate in the trunk area, and may spread to other sites, particularly in cases involving pruritic conditions. In chronic cases, most of the skin may be involved.

The initial characteristic sign of superficial bacterial folliculitis is an inflammatory papule (Fig. 15) or pustule (Fig. 16) that usually covers a follicle. In a recent study in which a model of superficial canine pyoderma was developed, the authors reported that papules can appear 24 hours after experimental infection, and can rapidly progress to pustules and subsequently more severe lesions in 48 to 96 hours. Pustules progress to crusts and epidermal collarettes (Fig. 17), and in some cases purulent exudate is observed 1 week after inoculation.

Epidermal collarettes may not be present in all forms of superficial bacterial folliculitis. Recent findings suggest that epidermal collaretes in exfoliative superficial pyoderma may have unique clinical and histological features, which differ from those of collaretes in impetigo and superficial bacterial folliculitis. It is possible that as-yet-unidentified toxins secreted by *S. pseudintermedius* can cause detachment or separation of the epidermis, giving rise to collarettes.

In short-haired breeds, raised nodules that resemble urticaria lesions may be observed (Fig. 18). These nodules give way to small, circular alopecia lesions as the hair falls out of the infected follicles. In dark-skinned breeds, these lesions may be confused with those of other aetiologies.

With progression, these alopecic lesions can merge, lending the patient's haircoat a classic "moth-eaten" appearance (Fig. 19), which is frequently confused with dermatophytosis (Fig. 20), among other diseases.

Lesion examination is more difficult in long-haired breeds, and often the initial signs of papules or pustules go unnoticed unless a thorough dermatological examination is performed. In general, the lesions that develop and are observed by both the owner and the veterinary surgeon are scaling, crusts, and, as the initial lesions progress, alopecia.

It should be noted that in both in short- and long-haired breeds the presence of intact pustules is uncommon, owing to their fragility. If observed, cytology of the lesion contents is recommended.

Superficial folliculitis in cats is rare and the most common presentation is a papular/crusting eruption, also known as miliary dermatitis, which is not easily distinguished from other crusted lesions in this species (Fig. 21). Areas of alopecia, scaling, and crusts on the head and neck, features more common to demodicosis or dermatophytosis, may be observed in some cats.

## Diagnostic findings

Diagnosis is based on the characteristic clinical signs and follicular involvement, in addition to cytological findings. However, it should be noted that pyoderma is usually a clinical sign secondary to an underlying disease, which must be identified and treated to avoid possible recurrence. Therefore, skin scraping and dermatophyte detection techniques can be of assistance in these cases.

Cytology may reveal neutrophilic inflammation with varying degrees of degeneration, as well as phagocytosed cocci (see Figs. 16b and 19b). If there is no exudate or if cytology reveals a bacterial distribution suggestive of another follicular inflammatory condition, additional tests (e.g. biopsy) should be performed.

Because bacterial folliculitis can clinically resemble other diseases, such as dermatophytosis, cytology should be performed in all suspected cases.

Histology may reveal neutrophilic exudate within the follicles (luminal suppurative folliculitis), in which bacteria may or may not be present. In samples obtained from chronic nonpustular lesions, suppurative superficial interstitial dermatitis, perifolliculitis, perifollicular fibrosis, and/or intraepidermal neutrophilic microabscesses may be observed. In the English Bulldog, the predominant lesions are marked superficial and follicular hyperkeratosis and interstitial inflammation around the adnexa (sebaceous gland, etc.).

## Therapeutic management

Topical and/or systemic treatment for 21 to 28 days is usually necessary to eliminate the infection. In case of recurrence, the underlying cause must be identified and corrected. If no response is observed after 2 weeks of treatment, a bacterial culture should be performed to evaluate the possibility of bacterial resistance.

Treatments for superficial bacterial folliculitis are discussed in Chapters 6 and 7.

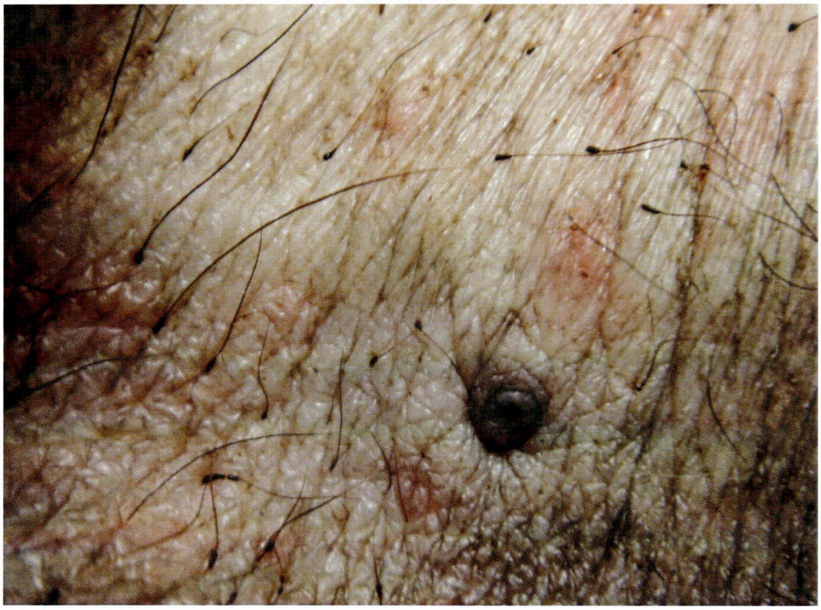

**Figure 15.** Superficial bacterial folliculitis: initial papular lesions covering one or more follicles are evident.

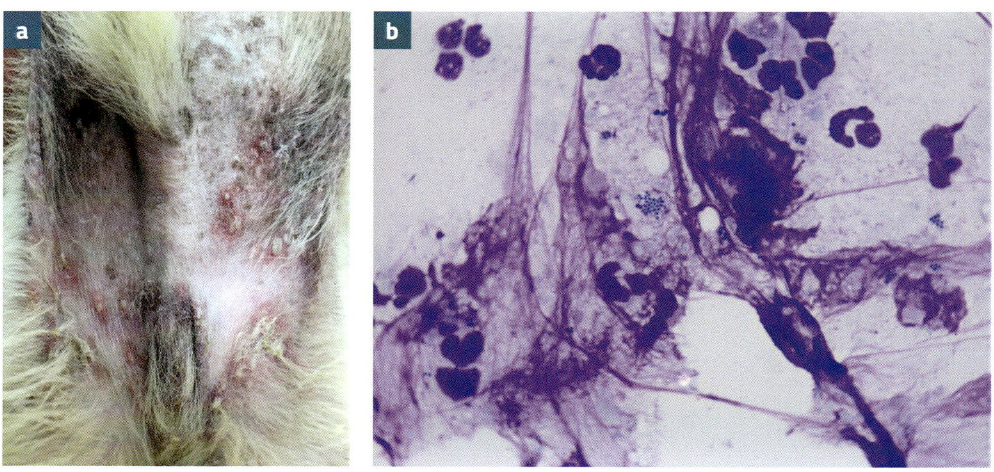

**Figure 16.** Superficial bacterial folliculitis. (a) Abdominal pustular lesions. (b) Cytology of the same lesions reveals neutrophilic inflammation with the presence of phagocytosed cocci and remnants of nuclear material.

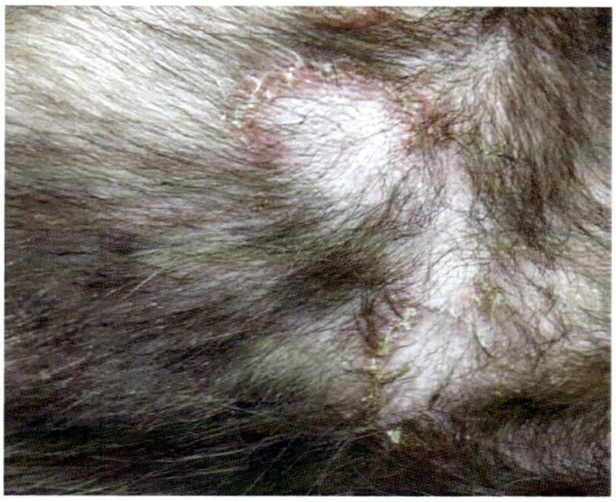

**Figure 17.** Epidermal collarettes in a patient with superficial pyoderma.

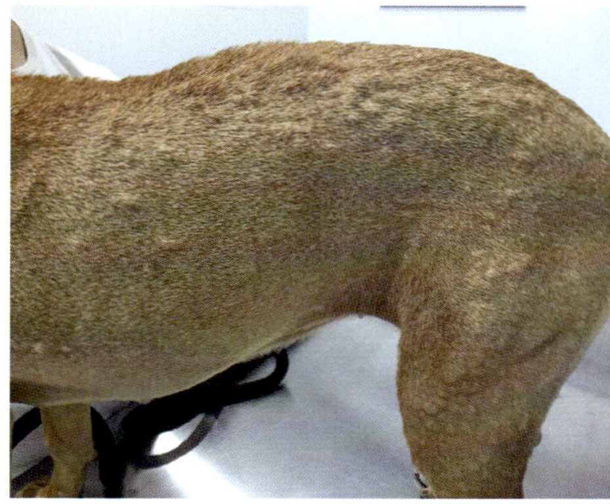

**Figure 18.** Early superficial bacterial folliculitis lesions. These raised nodules can be confused with urticaria lesions.

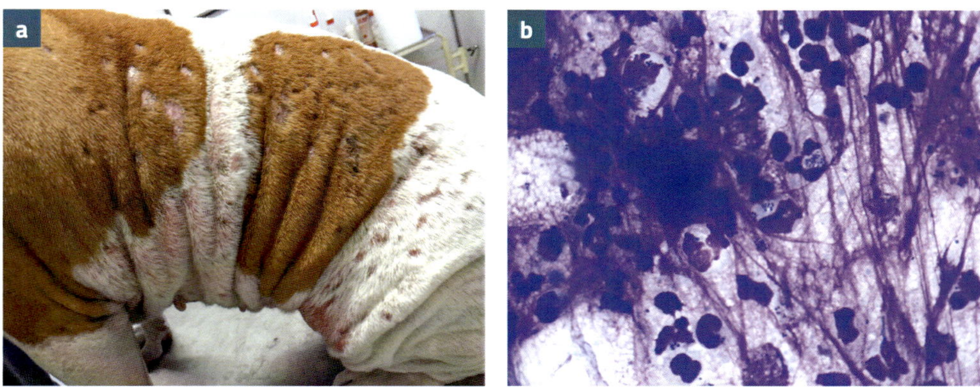

**Figure 19.** Superficial bacterial folliculitis. (a) Patient with a characteristic moth-eaten haircoat. (b) Cytology of the same patient reveals cocci and evidence of phagocytosis and marked inflammation.

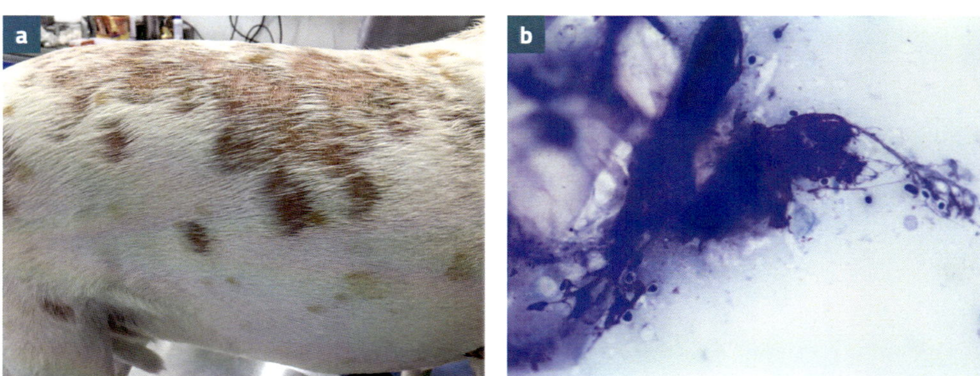

**Figure 20.** Dermatophytosis. (a) Alopecic lesions that lend the haircoat a moth-eaten appearance. (b) Cytology of the same patient showing evidence of arthrospores and organisms compatible with dermatophytes.

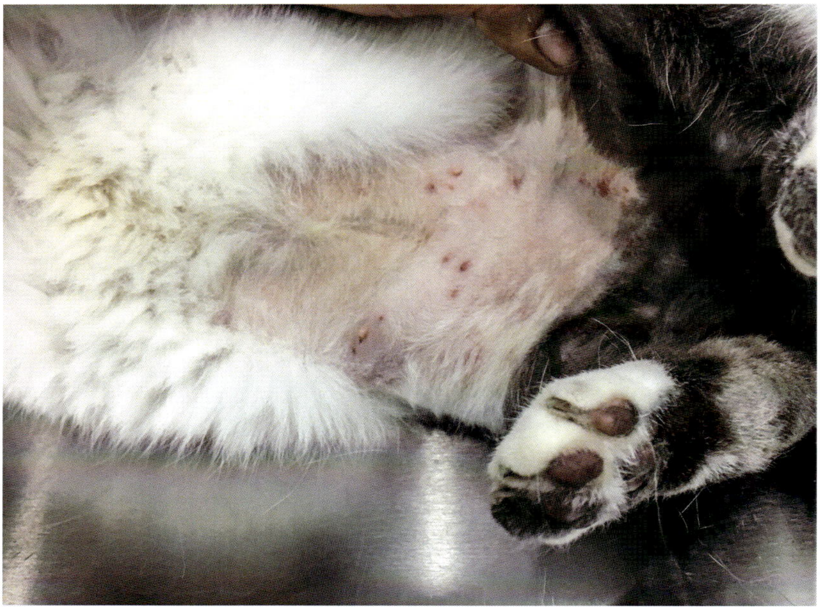

**Figure 21.** Miliary dermatitis in a cat. Note the linear papular lesions.

## SUMMARY

- Cytology is fundamental in cases of suspected bacterial infection.
- The most superficial bacterial infections can be treated with topical antibiotics, without the need for systemic treatment.
- Superficial bacterial infections have an underlying cause that must be identified and corrected.
- Several diseases can give rise to lesions characteristic of superficial bacterial folliculitis. Therefore, it is important to follow the steps of the diagnostic process and perform basic dermatological tests to avoid errors.

03

# DEEP BACTERIAL INFECTIONS

Deep bacterial infections and deep pyoderma affect tissues deeper than the hair follicle, which is often destroyed in the process. They can affect subcutaneous tissue, cause systemic signs of disease, and leave scarring lesions depending on the severity and depth of tissue damage.

Like surface and superficial pyoderma, deep pyoderma is usually linked to an underlying cause, which must be identified and corrected in order to control the secondary deep infection.

Possible causes of deep pyoderma affecting a small area include external trauma such as laceration or perforation, bites, and foreign bodies. In the case of more generalised lesions or those affecting the entire body, potential primary causes include systemic, parasitic, and opportunistic infectious diseases (Fig. 1).

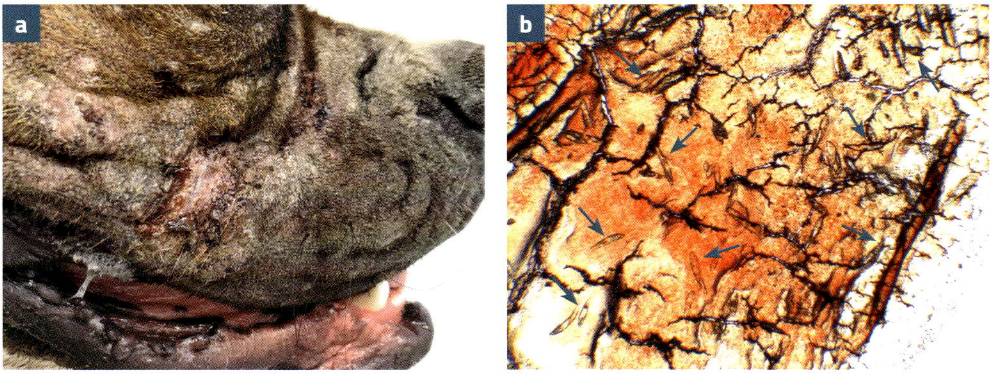


**Figure 1.** Generalised demodicosis in a dog. (a) Deep pyoderma with draining tracts. (b) Unstained smear of suppurative material containing mites of the genus *Demodex*.

In many cases, deep infections are the result of the evolution of a superficial infection, which progresses to and penetrates the deepest layers of the follicle (Fig. 2). This causes rupture of the follicular wall and subsequent furunculosis, which in turn causes the inflammation and infection to spread to the dermis and subcutaneous tissues (Fig. 3). This same infection spreads through different skin layers, advancing towards the surface, causing external fistulas and the formation of draining or suppurative tracts. It can also spread to deeper planes causing cellulitis and panniculitis.

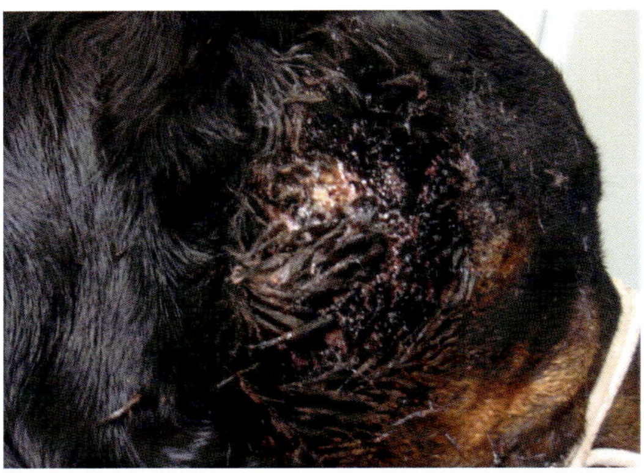

**Figure 2.** Deep pyotraumatic dermatitis before clipping.

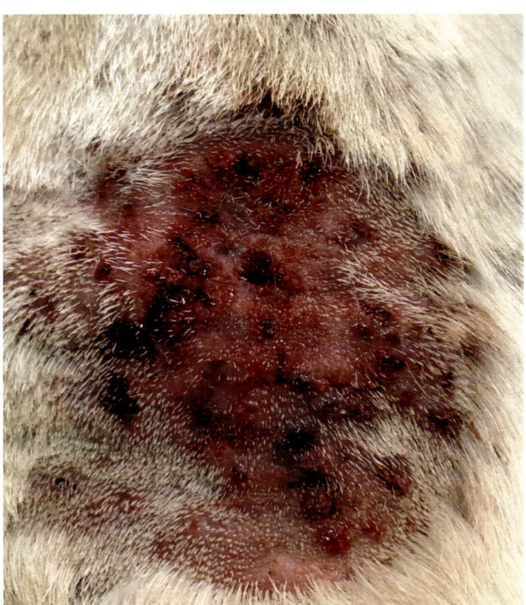

**Figure 3.** Deep pyotraumatic dermatitis after clipping. Furunculosis lesions, characterised by satellite papules, are evident.

The following factors predispose patients to deep pyoderma:

- Immunocompromise
- Severe damage to the follicle caused by a primary disease (e.g. demodicosis)
- Trauma (pressure, licking, scratching) in the affected area
- Inappropriate or ineffective treatment of a superficial infection
- Excessive administration of corticosteroids

## Skin lesions

Skin lesions include papulonodular lesions, nodules, plaques, haemorrhagic pustules, fistulas or draining tracts, and ulcers (Figs. 1–4).

Most conditions associated with deep pyoderma (deep folliculitis, furunculosis, cellulitis, subcutaneous abscesses) share similar pathogenic mechanisms.

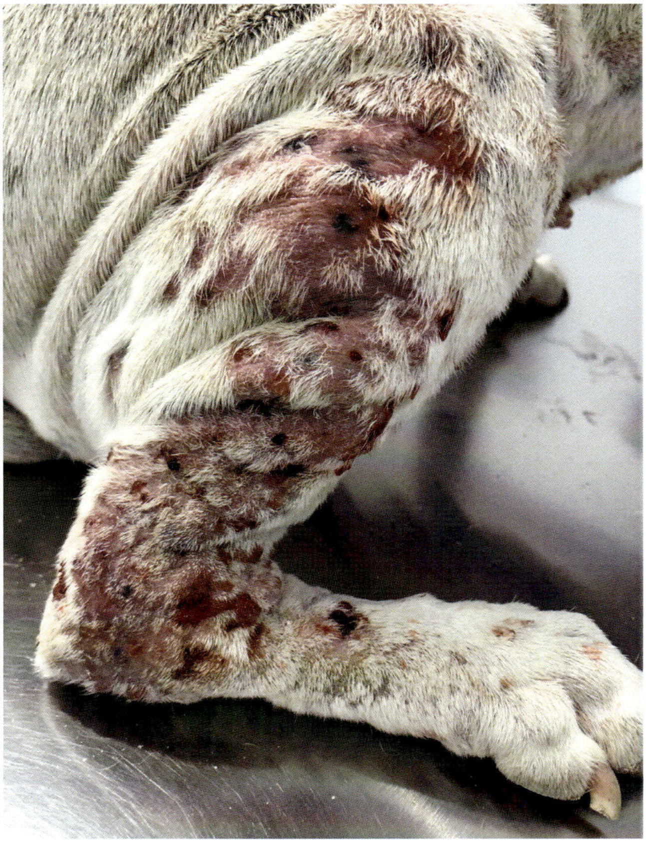

**Figure 4.** Bull Terrier with furunculosis complicated by solar dermatitis. Draining tracts can be observed.

## Sampling and cytological findings

As for most dermatoses, cytology is an invaluable tool for the diagnosis and evaluation of the inflammation of the patient's skin. It is recommended to clean the surface of the lesion with alcohol or an antiseptic solution before collecting samples from draining tracts. Next, pressure should be applied to the periphery of the lesion or a swab introduced into the draining tract in order to obtain a deeper sample and avoid contamination with superficial bacteria, which can lead to an incorrect diagnosis.

Once the sample has been obtained, it is spread on a slide, stained, and cytologically evaluated.

An understanding of the pathophysiology of deep pyoderma is required for correct interpretation of the cytological findings.

It is very common to observe neutrophilic inflammation with the presence of macrophages. The neutrophils do not show marked degeneration and the cytoplasm of macrophages can vary in size and shape. The cytoplasm can be vacuolated and contain amorphous material or remnants of leukocytes, which are phagocytosed by macrophages (Fig. 5).

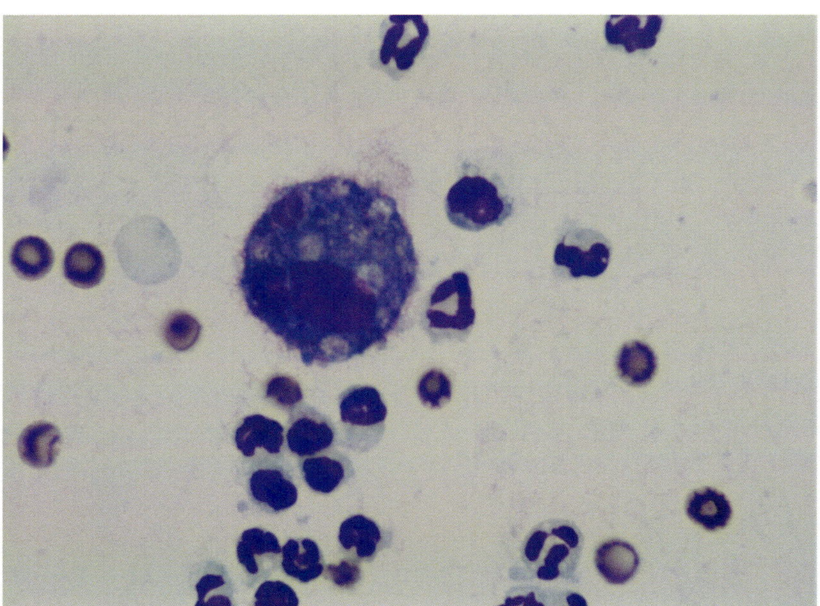

**Figure 5.** Macrophage phagocytosing neutrophils.

Rupture of the follicular wall results in the release and dissemination not only of microorganisms and inflammatory cells, but also follicular keratin and hair fragments, which act as foreign bodies and generate a pyogranulomatous reaction in which epithelioid macrophages and multinucleated or histiocytic giant cells are commonly found (Figs. 6 and 7). In cytological preparations these cells are often observed surrounding fragments of keratin, keratinocytes, or hair.

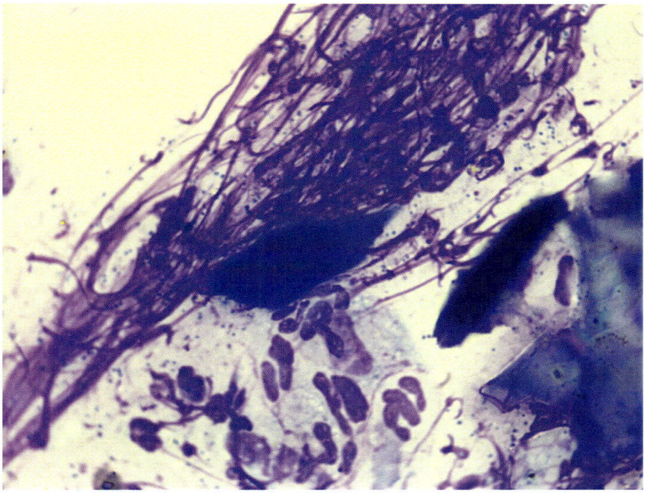

**Figure 6.** Neutrophilic/macrophagic inflammation with remnants of keratin and coccoid bacteria.

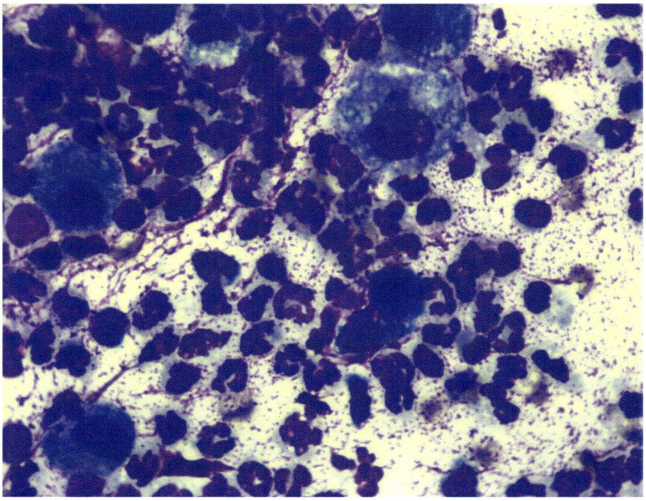

**Figure 7.** Pyogranulomatous inflammation.

A common finding in deep pyoderma cytology is the presence of fewer bacteria than in superficial or surface pyoderma. This is because the reaction to keratin generates intense inflammation, which dilutes the number of bacteria originally present in the follicle.

The possibility of infection should not be excluded even if bacteria are not detected in deep pyoderma cytology. However, the detection of a small number of bacteria is sufficient to confirm a diagnosis of deep infection.

Coccoid (*Staphylococcus* spp., *Streptococcus* spp.) or bacillus (*Pseudomonas, Proteus*) bacteria may be observed directly in the deep dermis or in the subcutaneous tissue (e.g. in cases of bites or foreign body contamination).

Other findings in deep pyoderma cytology include erythrocytes, eosinophils, and, in the most chronic cases, reactive fibroblasts and the presence of lymphoplasmacytes.

## Folliculitis, deep furunculosis, and cellulitis

Folliculitis, deep furunculosis, and cellulitis can begin as bacterial, fungal, or parasitic follicular infections. Other causes include adverse drug reaction, endocrine abnormalities, seborrhoea, and immunosuppression.

The most commonly implicated bacterium is *Staphylococcus pseudintermedius,* but *Proteus* spp., *Pseudomonas* spp., and *Escherichia coli* are also commonly observed.

Histopathological examination of biopsy samples can be useful to understand the mechanism, aetiology, and stage of progression of folliculitis and furunculosis. Folliculitis associated with bacteria, fungi, or parasites is usually suppurative in the early stages. In cases associated with atopic dermatitis, allergies, or seborrheic dermatitis, folliculitis is usually spongiotic and mononuclear, whereas chronic folliculitis can become granulomatous or pyogranulomatous, especially if furunculosis develops.

The nature of the lesions will depend largely on the extent of the follicular area involved, as well as the depth and severity of the process.

## Furunculosis

Furunculosis is a form of deep folliculitis in which the follicle ruptures and microorganisms, keratin, and inflammatory cells are released into the dermis.

Regardless of the cause, furunculosis is associated with tissue eosinophilia due to foreign body reactions in response to hairs or free keratin. When there is eosinophilia secondary to infectious furunculosis, intraluminal and intramural neutrophils predominate and are found in numbers equivalent to those of eosinophils in perifollicular dermal inflammation. The predominance of eosinophils in all these locations suggests a noninfectious aetiology. The absence of eosinophils in tissue affected by furunculosis is most commonly associated with immunosuppression (especially in patients receiving long-term glucocorticoid therapy) and demodicosis.

### Skin lesions

Macroscopically, furunculosis is characterised by an intense red, occasionally painful, erythematous nodular lesion, which fistulises after a few days, secreting bloody fluid and giving rise to draining tracts.

### Diagnostic findings

Examination of cytological preparations of the secreted material reveals macrophagic and neutrophilic inflammation, which can appear pyogranulomatous owing to the intense reaction directed at the foreign material in the dermis. The causative or complicating microorganisms may be visible, but in most cases are not easily detected. Therefore, the absence of microorganisms in deep infection cytology does not completely rule out their presence.

Histology may reveal follicular rupture with neutrophilic and macrophagic infiltrate surrounding the lesion.

### Therapeutic management

Although uncommon in most cases of deep pyoderma, patients should be monitored for sepsis. Failure to achieve resolution in these cases is primarily due to failure to identify the primary cause. The primary cause should be corrected while controlling the secondary infection, the treatment of which can take up to 6 weeks. Most cases resolve after 21 days of treatment.

The choice of a systemic antimicrobial treatment should be based on the cytological and bacterial culture findings, applying the principles of rational antibiotic use, as discussed in Chapter 8.

Systemic treatment can be combined with topical antimicrobial therapy.

## Abscesses

An abscess is a subcutaneous cavity that contains pus and is usually surrounded by a reactive border. In most cases abscesses form as a result of bites, scratches, or puncture with a foreign body.

## Skin lesions

The first lesion to appear is a nodule or mass with a fluctuating appearance that eventually fistulises towards the skin, releasing purulent or bloody material. Upon palpation the mass may be hotter than the rest of the body.

## Diagnostic findings

Cytology is nonspecific and may reveal neutrophils and macrophages. Erythrocytes and fibrin filaments may also be present. Occasionally, the causative agents (filamentous or coccoid bacteria) and active phagocytosis may be evident (Figs. 8 and 9).

Histology may reveal inflammatory cells (neutrophils and macrophages) obscured by granulation tissue.

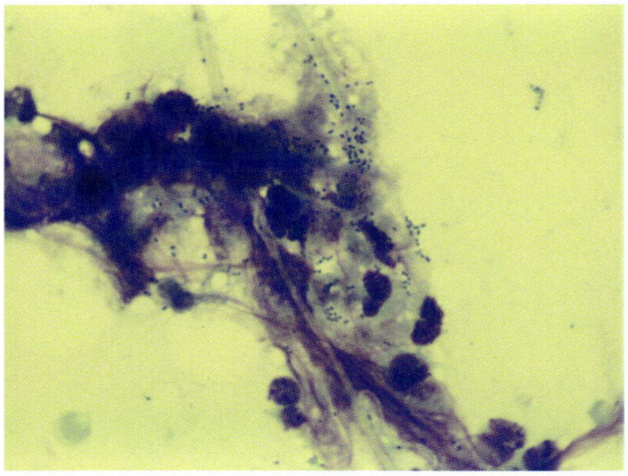

**Figure 8.** Cytology of an abscess. Note the neutrophilic degradation and phagocytosis of cocci.

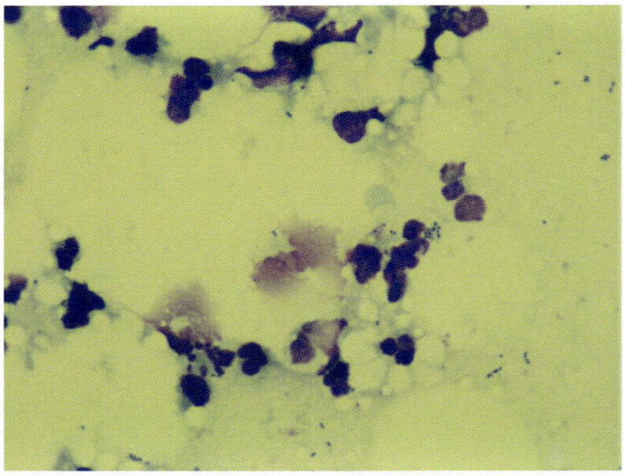

**Figure 9.** Cytology of an abscess showing phagocytosis of cocci with neutrophil degeneration.

## Therapeutic management

The lesions and the material within the abscess should be drained and, if necessary, the affected tissue should be debrided and the surrounding area cleaned.

Therapeutic management should be accompanied by antibiotic treatment specific for the microorganisms involved. The choice of antimicrobial agent can be based on the cytological findings or, for greater specificity, the results of the culture and antibiotic sensitivity test.

In the case of intact cats, castration is recommended to prevent abscesses caused by fights.

## Cellulitis

Cellulitis is characterised by the spread of an infectious process to deeper layers of the skin, and can be severe (Fig. 10). The infectious and/or inflammatory material is poor in bacterial content and the lesions extend laterally to affect the adjacent tissue.

## Skin lesions

Cellulitis can cause oedema, which results in friable tissue with a dark, devitalised appearance. Tissue may detach if large areas are affected.

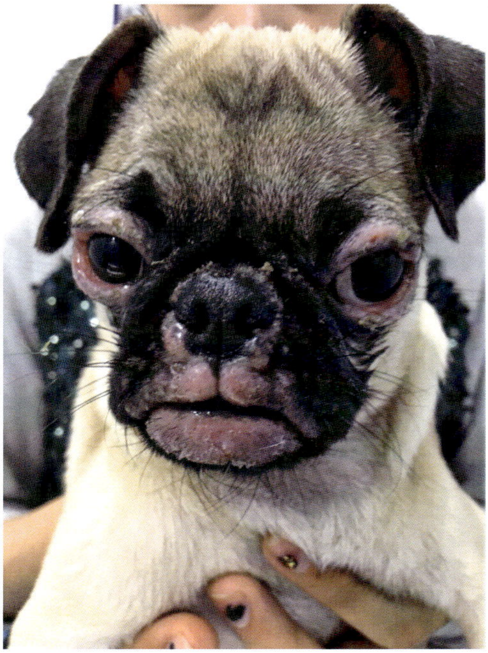

**Figure 10.** Juvenile cellulitis in a Pug.

### Diagnostic findings

It is important to try to identify the microorganisms involved and to treat the patient based on the results of cytology or culture.

The cytological findings do not differ greatly from those of furunculosis, and reveal large amounts of neutrophils and macrophages, and (in some cases) the causative agent. Phagocytosis of neutrophils by macrophages may be observed, as well as inflammatory reactions caused by the presence of keratin or necrotic tissue material.

### Therapeutic management

The therapeutic management of cellulitis is the same as that indicated for deep pyoderma and/or furunculosis.

## Mycobacterial infections

Table 1 summarises the most common mycobacterial infections, their clinical characteristics, and the corresponding diagnostic approach (Figs. 11–14).

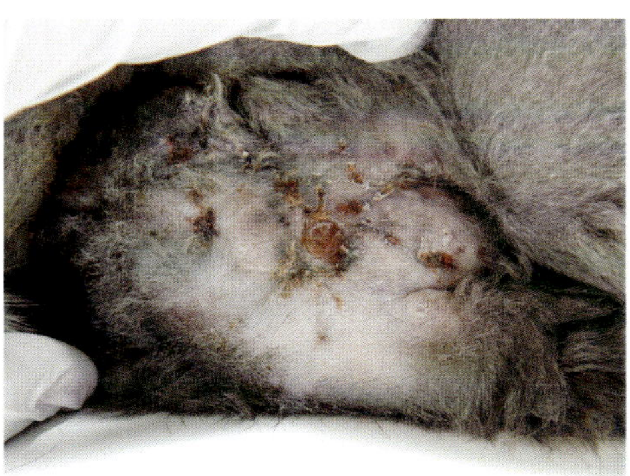

**Figure 11.** Abdominal lesions in a cat with mycobacterial infection. Image courtesy of Elizabeth Layne (DVM, DACVD).

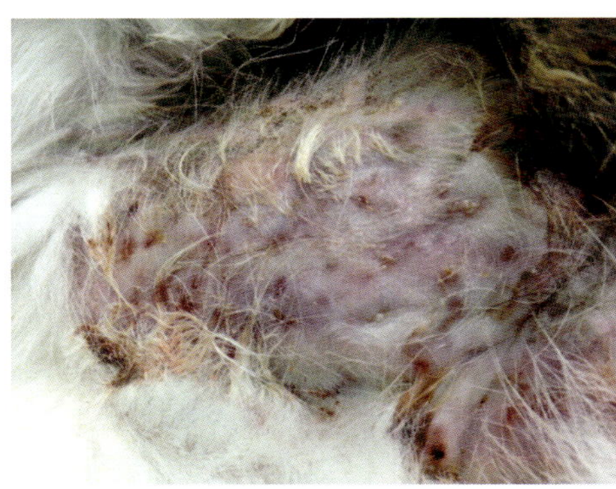

**Figure 12.** Atypical feline mycobacteriosis. Image courtesy of Joe Bernstein (DVM, DACVD).

Table 1. Most common infections caused by mycobacteria.

<table>
<tr><th>Diseases and causal agents</th><th>Characteristics</th><th>Clinical signs</th><th>Diagnosis</th></tr>
<tr><td>■ Tuberculosis (caused by Mycobacterium tuberculosis complex, M. bovis, and M. microti)<br>■ Feline leprosy (caused by M. lepraemurium)</td><td>Caused by obligate mycobacterial parasites in immunocompromised animals.<br>Can be localised or generalised.</td><td rowspan="4">■ Multiple or solitary nodules, plaques, abscesses, or ulcers may appear on the skin or in subcutaneous tissue<br>■ Thick, foul-smelling, greenish-yellow discharge<br>■ Patients with anorexia, fever, weight loss, localised or generalised lymphadenopathy<br>■ Feline leprosy: focal mass with subcutaneous granuloma, fistula or abscess formation, regional lymphadenomegaly</td><td rowspan="4">■ Clinical history<br>■ Physical examination<br>■ Radiographic examination<br>■ Cytology with Ziehl-Neelsen staining or staining for acid-fast organisms<br>■ Biopsy<br>■ Culture<br>■ Serological test<br>■ Lymphocyte blastogenesis test<br>■ Bacillus Calmette–Guérin test<br>■ Purified protein derivative test</td></tr>
<tr><td>■ Leproid granuloma (as-yet unidentified agents, different species of mycobacteria)</td><td>Localised disease caused by a saprophytic mycobacterium in immunocompromised animals. Lesions are self-limiting.</td></tr>
<tr><td>■ Panniculitis caused by mycobacteria (M. smegmatis, M. fortiutum, M. chelonae)<br>■ Localised skin infections (M. avium)</td><td>Localised disease caused by a saprophytic mycobacterium in immunocompromised animals. Lesions are located the hypodermis.</td></tr>
<tr><td>■ M. avium (young adult Abyssinian cats)<br>■ M. genavense (ferrets and cats with FIV)<br>■ Feline leprosy in older cats</td><td>Disseminated disease caused by mycobacteria in immunodeficient patients.</td></tr>
</table>

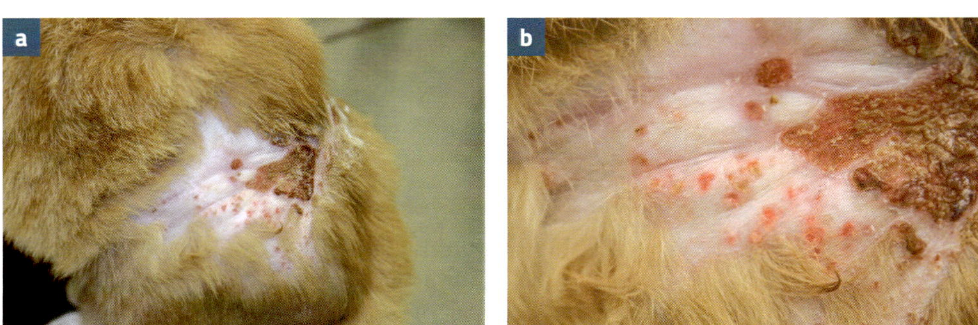


Figure 13. Atypical feline mycobacteriosis. (a) Note the central and peripheral lesions. (b) Magnified image of lesions. Note the thickened, crusted ulcerative lesion. Images courtesy of Candace Sousa (DVM, DACVD).

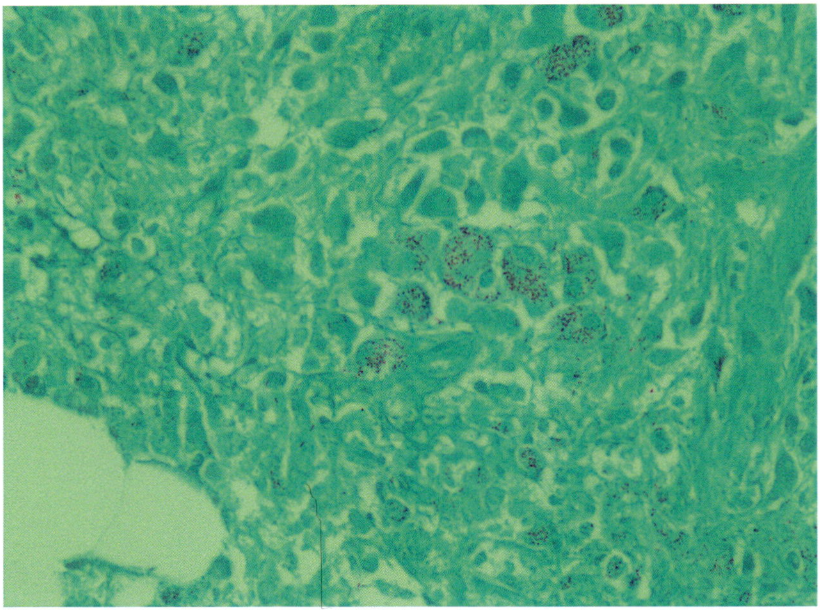

**Figure 14.** Histopathological section of leproid granuloma. Note the filamentous organisms. Image courtesy of Elizabeth Layne (DVM, DACVD).

## Therapeutic management

Infections caused by mycobacteria require prolonged treatments with antibiotics (doxycycline, quinolones, and clarithromycin), selected in accordance with the findings of the bacterial culture and antibiotic sensitivity test. Surgical excision is recommended in cases in which a large amount of tissue is affected.

> Antibiotic therapy should be continued for 4–6 weeks after clinical cure.

## Treatment of leproid granuloma

The treatment of leproid granuloma consists of surgical excision of individual lesions. Severe or refractory cases are treated using a combination of rifampicin (10–15 mg/kg) and clarithromycin (15–25 mg/kg administered in 2 to 3 doses per day). Clarithromycin can be substituted with doxycycline (5–10 mg/kg twice daily). Liver function should be monitored during treatment.

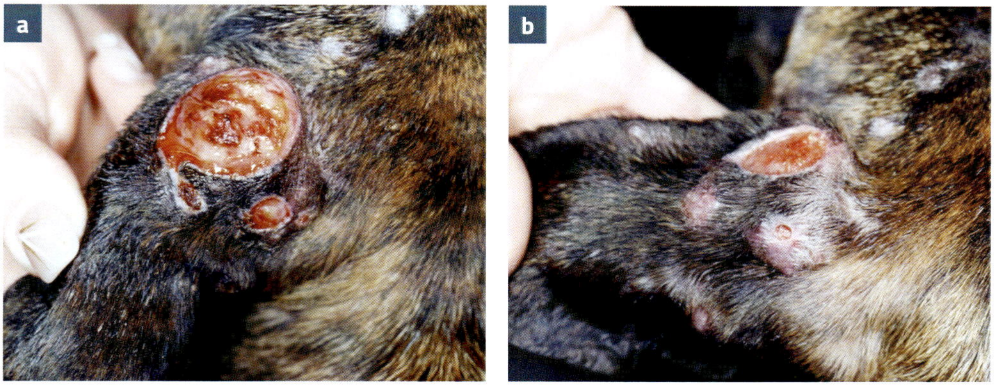


**Figure 15.** Leproid granuloma on a dog's ear. Appearance of the lesions (a) before and (b) 2 weeks after treatment. Images courtesy of Candace Sousa (DVM, DACVD).

### Treatment of feline leprosy

Surgical excision is recommended in cases involving localised lesions. Systemic therapy consists of combinations of 2 or 3 antimicrobial agents. Clofazimine (10 mg/kg once per day, or 25–50 mg every 1 or 2 days) is effective for the treatment of *M. lepraemurium*. It can be combined with clarithromycin (62.5 mg twice daily) or rifampicin (10–15 mg/kg once daily). Treatment should be continued for 2 months after clinical resolution.

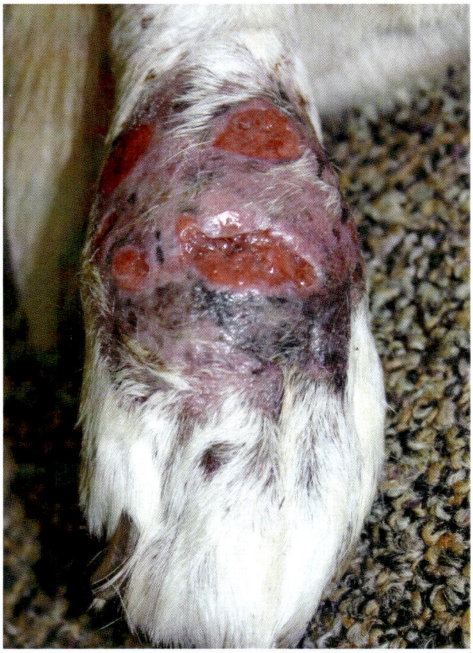

## Actinomycosis

Actinomycosis is a rare pyogranulomatous or suppurative disease caused by different species of bacteria of the genus *Actinomyces* (Fig. 16). These bacteria are gram-positive, catalase-positive, non-acid-fast filamentous bacilli. These opportunistic, anaerobic bacteria reside in the oral cavity and intestine.

Infection with these organisms occurs as a result of trauma or contamination of penetrating wounds, particularly those that may contain foreign bodies. The disease can develop between 2 months and 2 years after infection.

**Figure 16.** Actinomycosis in a Labrador Retriever. Image courtesy of Candace Sousa (DVM, DACVD).

## Skin lesions

The most characteristic lesion is inflammation or a subcutaneous abscess on the head, neck, thorax, or abdominal or paralumbar region (Fig. 17). The lesion is usually mild and may contain draining tracts. Paralumbar lesions may develop as a consequence of retroperitoneal involvement.

If draining tracts are present a yellow-grey discharge with haemorrhagic exudate, sometimes containing yellow sulphur granules, is observed.

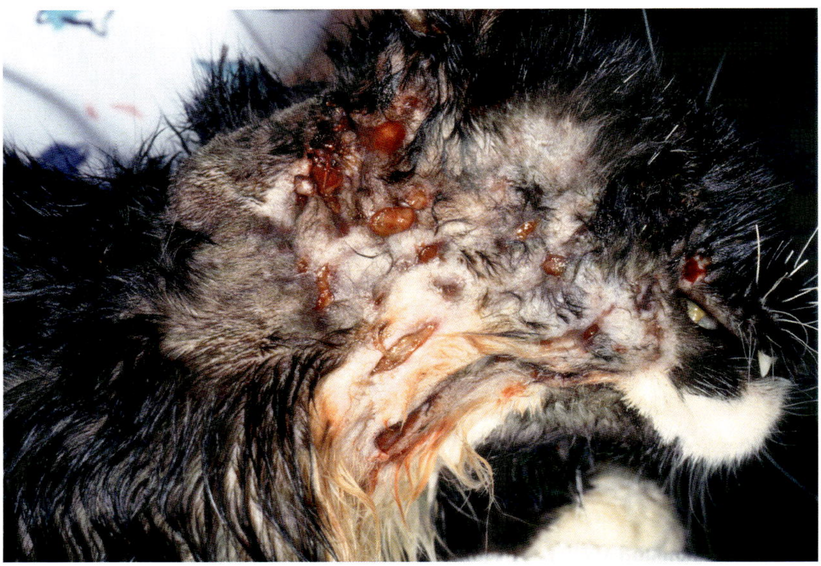

**Figure 17.** Actinomycosis in a cat. Image courtesy of Candace Sousa (DVM, DACVD).

## Diagnostic findings

Diagnosis is established based on the results of anaerobic culture, which can take 2 to 4 weeks, although the filamentous bacilli may be visible in cytological preparations (obtained by aspiration or direct impression) of the secreted material.

Histology reveals nodular to diffuse dermatitis, panniculitis, and pyogranulomatous inflammation. Tissue granules or sulphur granules are present in about half of all cases.

### Therapeutic management

Treatment may include surgical excision or debridement of the lesion, along with long-term treatment with systemic antibiotics (e.g. penicillin). Clindamycin, erythromycin, chloramphenicol, tetracyclines, and cephalosporins can be useful in certain cases. Treatment should be continued for at least 1 month after remission. Relapse can occur in some cases.

## Nocardiosis

Nocardiosis is a rare disease characterised by pyogranulomatous and suppurative infection of the skin or lungs that can spread to other regions. It is caused by *Nocardia* spp. These bacteria are partially acid-fast.

### Skin lesions

This disease is indistinguishable from actinomycosis; cellulitis lesions, ulcerated nodules, abscesses, and draining tracts can be observed in affected patients. It commonly affects damaged areas of skin, especially on the limbs, and may be associated with regional lymphadenomegaly.

Affected cats often present with abdominal lesions that resemble those of panniculitis or mycobacterial infections (Fig. 18). Clinical signs include pyothorax together with anorexia, fever, depression, weakness, dyspnoea, and neurological signs.

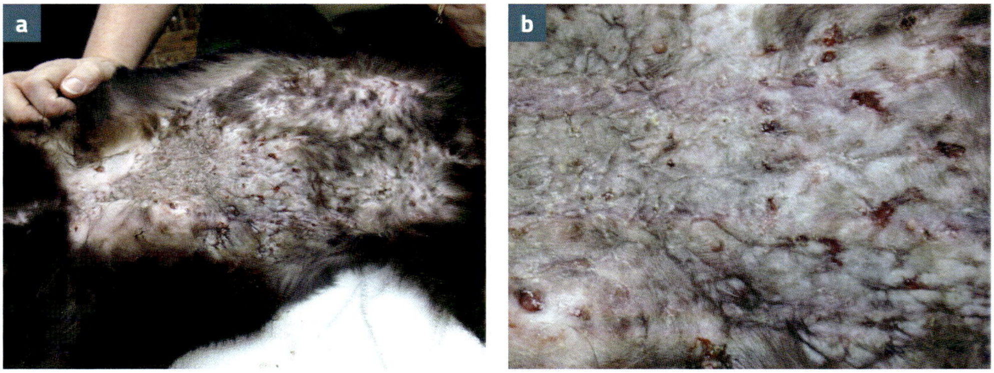


**Figure 18.** Nocardiosis. (a) Lesions on the abdomen of a cat. (b) Magnified view of the lesions. Images courtesy of Candace Sousa (DVM, DACVD).

## Diagnostic findings

Diagnosis of nocardiosis is based on cytology of a direct impression smear or aspirate of the nodules (Fig. 19). Histology may reveal diffuse nodular dermatitis, panniculitis, or both. Tissue granules may also be observed.

## Therapeutic management

Treatment includes drainage of the lesion along with antimicrobial therapy (clarithromycin, erythromycin, amikacin, trimethoprim–sulfamethoxazole, cefotaxime, imipenem, or minocycline). Where appropriate, antibiotic susceptibility studies should be carried out.

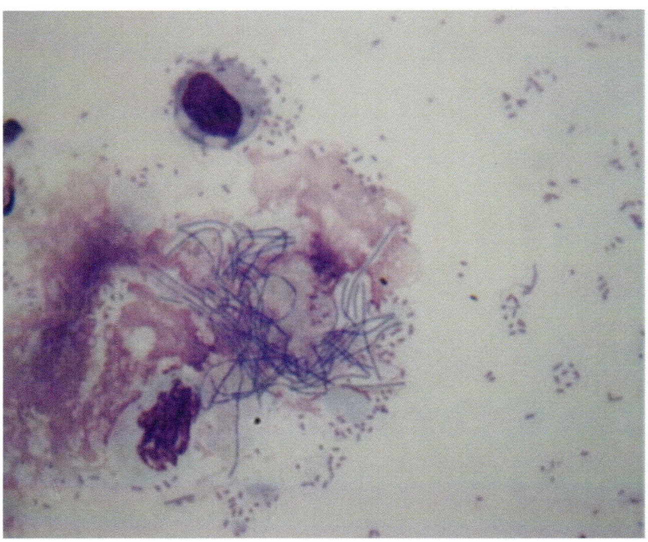

**Figure 19.** Cytology of nocardiosis. Note the presence of filamentous *Nocardia* spp. organisms. Image courtesy of Porfirio Trapala (DVM).

### SUMMARY

- Deep bacterial infections usually have an underlying cause that must be identified and corrected.
- Some organisms require special staining or more prolonged culture than those that cause superficial pyoderma.
- Although cytology may not enable identification of the causal agent, it can help guide the diagnosis by revealing the types of inflammatory cells present in the infection and the changes they undergo.

04

# PSEUDOPYODERMA

Pseudopyoderma refers to a group of diseases that clinically resemble pyoderma. Although their aetiology is distinct from that of pyoderma, these conditions can involve bacterial complications associated with inflammation.

The types of pseudopyoderma covered in this chapter are callus pyoderma, juvenile cellulitis, acne, and facial eosinophilic folliculitis and furunculosis.

## Callus pyoderma

Calluses are oval or round hyperkeratotic plaques that form at pressure points, particularly in areas of skin covering bony prominences (Figs. 1–3). They most often affect large-breed dogs that lie on cement, brick, or other hard surfaces. In some breeds, particularly those with a prominent thoracic cavity, calluses can appear on the chest.

They can also develop in unusual locations in patients who adopt specific positions due to certain orthopaedic conditions.

Histologically, a callus is an area of irregular or papillary epidermal hyperplasia with orthokeratotic to parakeratotic hyperkeratosis. Small follicular cysts may be observed in the dermis. Clinically, the lesions are hairless and have a wrinkled appearance.

**Management of this condition requires environmental measures; incidence can be reduced by providing animals with soft mattresses. However, in most cases pets either destroy or refuse to use this type of bedding.**

Soft elbow patches can be used to reduce the impact, although these are not tolerated by many patients, and are generally removed.

The prolonged presence of calluses and repeated trauma at the affected area results in epidermal rupture, ulceration at the pressure points, and fistulas. These lesions are very susceptible to secondary infection.

Infection is commonly caused by *Staphylococcus pseudintermedius*, although other secondary contaminants can be isolated.

Pressure in these areas can also result in penetration of the dermis by hair shafts, giving rise to a foreign body reaction and subsequent furunculosis or even cellulitis. It is common to observe hairs protruding from inside the callus when pressure is applied to the affected area.

Owing to the aforementioned pathophysiological process, cytology of pyogranulomatous inflammation often reveals large numbers of macrophages surrounding hair shafts or keratin particles.

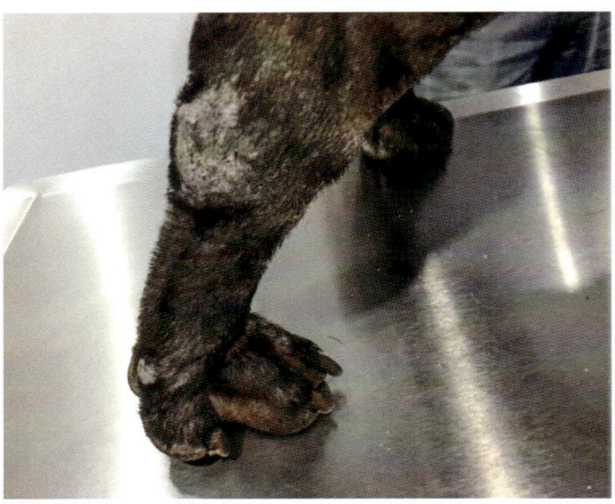

**Figure 1.** Callus formation and hyperkeratosis on the calcaneus.

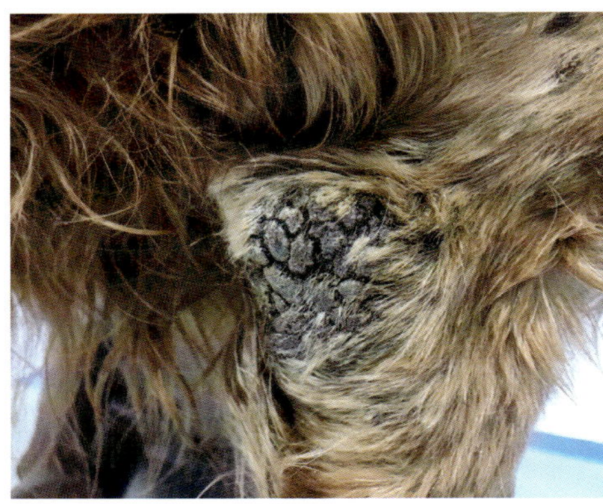

**Figure 2.** Callus on the elbow of a geriatric patient.

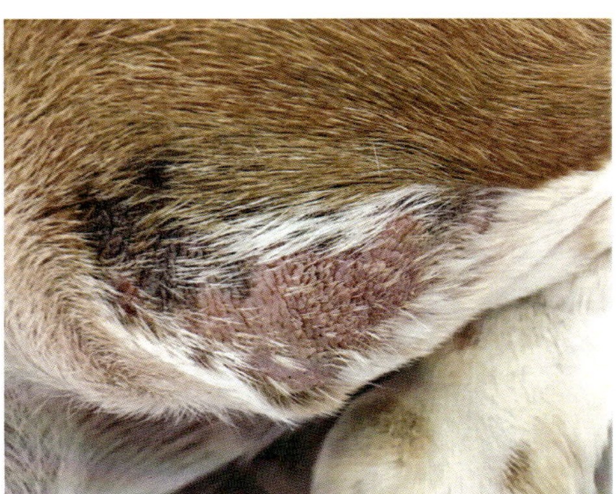

**Figure 3.** Hyperkeratosis and callus in the knee area of a patient with atopic dermatitis.

### Therapeutic management

Secondary bacterial infections should be treated for an average of 6 weeks, and cytologically evaluated every 15 days. In many cases it can be difficult for the owner to detect any improvement owing to the persistence of the primary lesion (callus).

The secondary infection should be treated while also administering treatments to soften the affected area and eliminate the callus.

Although recommended in some cases, surgical removal can result in post-operative complications and poor healing. Moreover, in many cases wound closure can occur by secondary intention, generating granulation tissue.

Keratolytic and keratoplastic products (particularly ointments) containing salicylic acid and sulphur may help to soften calluses. Some essential oils are also indicated for softening calluses. Magnesium salts may be beneficial in cases in which hairs are embedded in the lesion. Beneficial effects have also been attributed to haemorrhoid ointments containing shark liver oil and yeast extracts.

## Juvenile cellulitis

Also known as juvenile pyoderma or puppy strangles, this is a sterile inflammatory disease that affects puppies between 3 weeks and 4 months of age. Clinical signs include facial inflammation followed by the appearance of papules and pustules that can progress to crusted, draining tracts within about 48 hours.

Well-delimited lesions predominantly appear around the eyes and on the chin, and are accompanied by inflammation of the ear canals, in which cytology may reveal overgrowth of bacilli. The lesions can be painful. Consequently, this condition is sometimes mistaken for an infectious process (Figs. 4–11).

Corticosteroids at immunosuppressive doses are the treatment of choice. In general, lesions resolve within weeks of starting treatment. The dose of corticosteroids should be reduced as soon as clinical remission is achieved.

Once resolved, juvenile cellulitis tends not to recur. The aetiology of this condition remains unclear, although it is thought to involve regulatory immunological processes.

This disease can represent a challenge for clinicians without prior experience; resolution can be difficult to achieve given the lack of response to antibiotic treatment. Diagnosis is established based on histological findings and clinical signs.

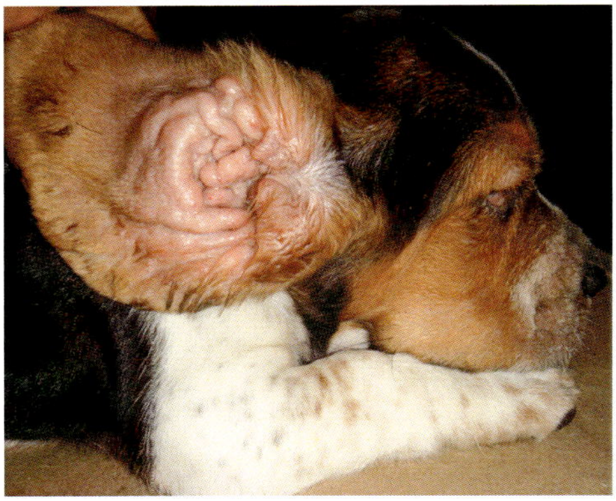

**Figure 4.** Otitis externa in a Beagle puppy with juvenile cellulitis.

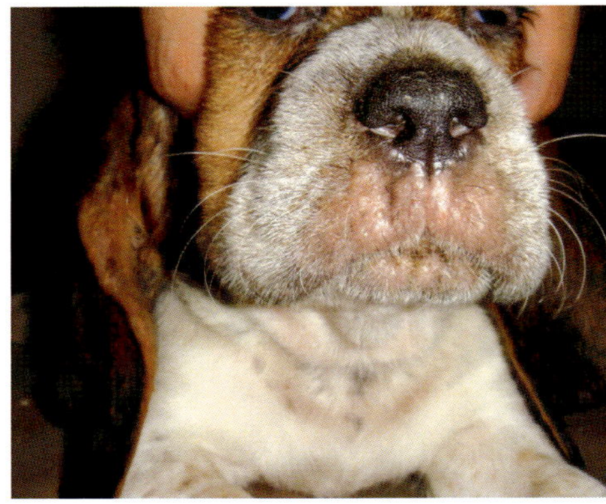

**Figure 5.** Lesions on the chin of the Beagle puppy from the previous image.

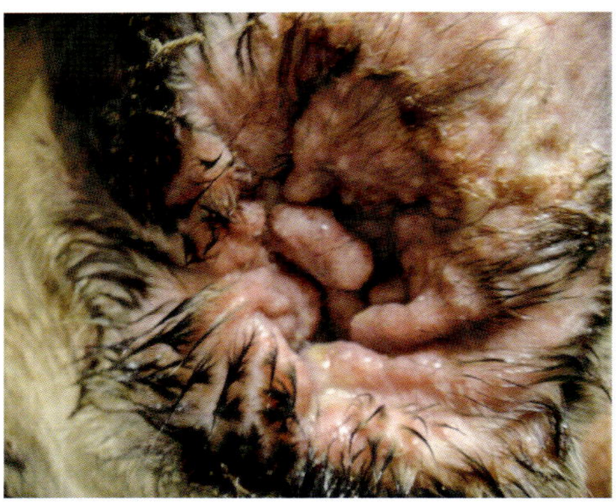

**Figure 6.** Otitis externa in a Mastiff puppy with juvenile cellulitis.

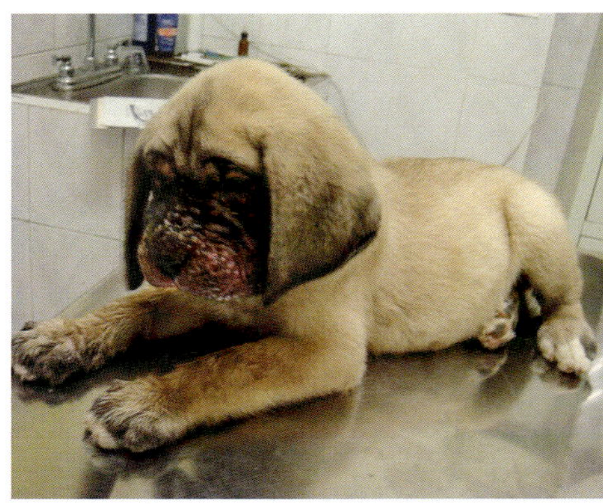

**Figure 7.** Facial lesions in the Mastiff puppy from the previous image.

## Acne

Acne is a keratinisation defect that can affect both dogs and cats and is mainly considered a follicular disorder. Examination of the lipid profile of the lipid material in comedones has revealed a primarily epidermal (rather than sebaceous) origin, suggesting that the sebaceous glands play a less important role than in humans.

In both dogs and cats, the typical lesions are papules and furuncles, which usually appear on the chin and lips, in some cases with secondary infection. In dogs, acne tends to be the result of trauma and follicular damage.

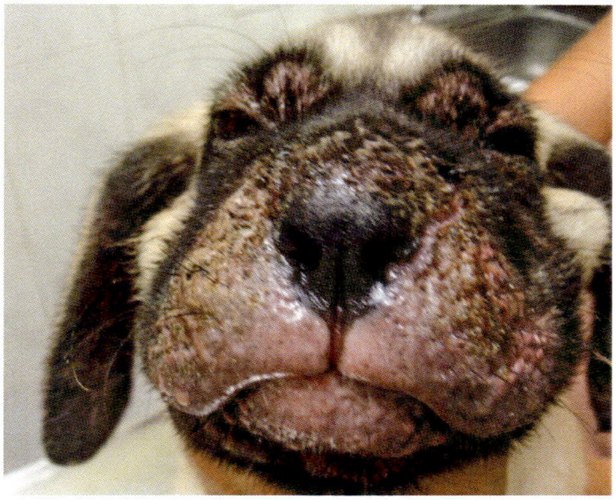

**Figure 8.** Cellulitis lesions and crusts on the chin of patient from the previous image.

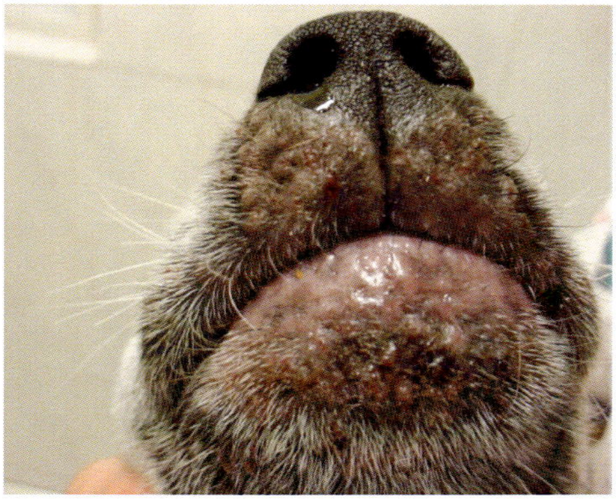

**Figure 9.** Papules and plaques on the chin of an Australian Shepherd with juvenile cellulitis.

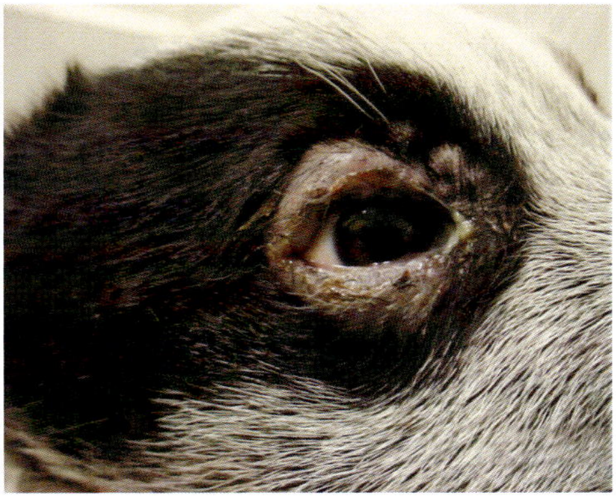

**Figure 10.** Periocular lesions in the patient from the previous image.

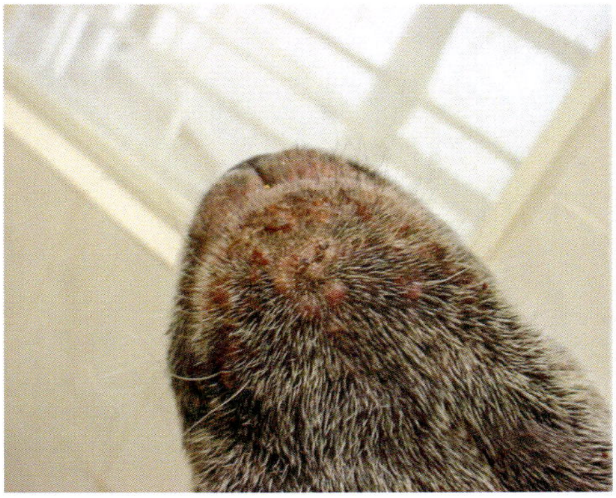

**Figure 11.** Papular lesions and crusts on the ventral area of the chin of the patient from the previous two images.

In cats, lesions tend to appear exclusively on the chin (Figs. 12 and 13). Some patients may experience a single episode throughout their life, while in others acne may constitute a recurrent problem.

Causes of feline acne include poor grooming habits, predisposition to seborrhoea, abnormal sebum production, hair cycle alterations, stress, and immunosuppression.

A hormonal influence appears unlikely, given that males and females are affected in equal proportions.

> Comedones around the chin and lips are the first lesions to appear, and can progress to papular and pustular lesions. Folliculitis, furunculosis, and suppurative cellulitis may develop in severe cases.

In cases in which acne is complicated by infectious processes, commonly isolated agents include β-haemolytic streptococci, *Pasteurella multocida*, *Staphylococcus*, *Malassezia*, and in some cases dermatophytes.

Diagnosis is based on examination of the lesions (Fig. 14). Cytology can be used to confirm or rule out the presence of specific microorganisms, and is thus of diagnostic value. A trichogram can be used to identify signs of keratinisation defects. Histological findings include keratosis and plugging and dilatation of the follicle in early stages. Perifolliculitis, folliculitis, and furunculosis with associated pyogranulcmatous dermatitis are observed in more advanced stages.

The treatment of feline and canine acne includes application of topical solutions for follicular cleansing and disinfection of the area. While benzoyl peroxide is useful as a follicular cleansing agent, it can cause irritation in some cats. The use of antiseptic wipes containing solutions such as chlorhexidine can be useful during the initial follicular phase. In cases of secondary infection, systemic therapy with antimicrobial agents may be required.

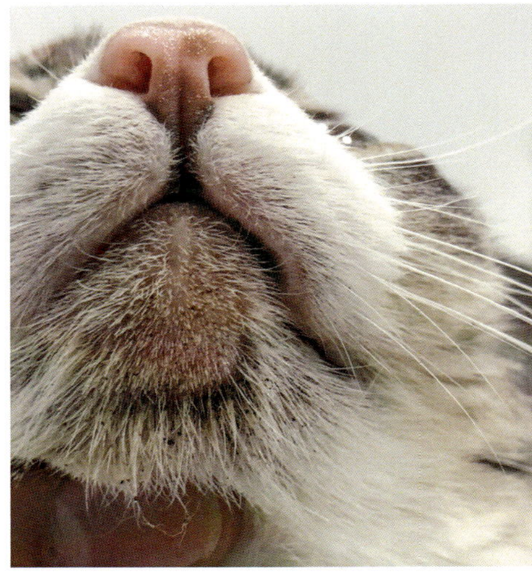

**Figure 12.** Comedones and alopecia in a cat with acne.

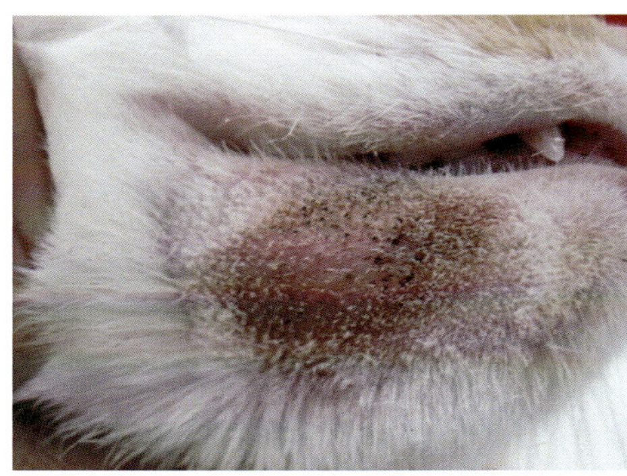

**Figure 13.** Comedones, alopecia, and erythema in a cat with acne.

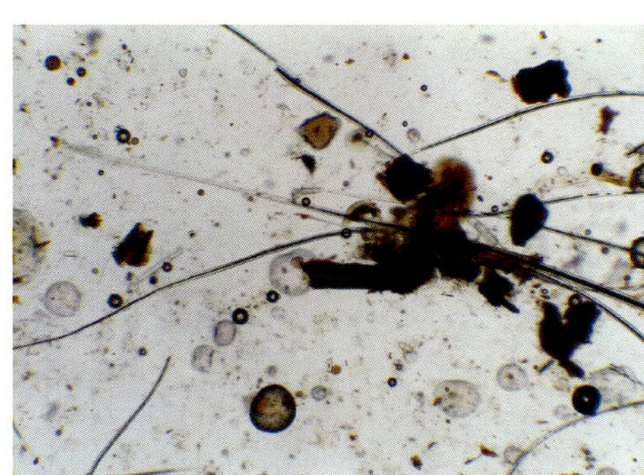

**Figure 14.** Trichogram of a cat with acne showing keratinous/sebaceous material and follicular casts.

## Facial folliculitis and eosinophilic furunculosis

This condition mainly affects the face. It is caused by a hypersensitivity reaction, which in some cases can be triggered by insects and other arthropods.

The associated lesions are nodules, papules, crusts and exudative lesions (Figs.15–18). In many cases the first lesions to appear are pruritic vesicles. The most commonly affected areas are the nasal bridge and chin. Clinical signs are usually absent, but can include fever, anorexia, and discomfort.

Diagnosis is easily established based on clinical signs and cytological findings. Cytology reveals eosinophilic inflammation, although in some cases degenerate neutrophils and cocci, with or without phagocytosis, are observed (Fig. 19).

Histology reveals the presence of infiltrative eosinophilic mural folliculitis, luminal folliculitis, and eosinophilic furunculosis.

Because folliculitis is caused by an underlying hypersensitivity reaction, patients respond rapidly to corticosteroid treatment. Secondary bacterial infection occurs in rare cases; depending on the cytological findings antimicrobial therapy may be required in these cases.

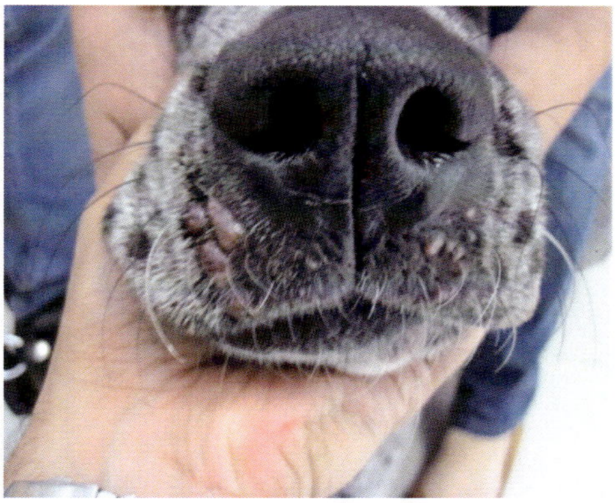

**Figure 15.** Eosinophilic furunculosis on the chin of a Great Dane.

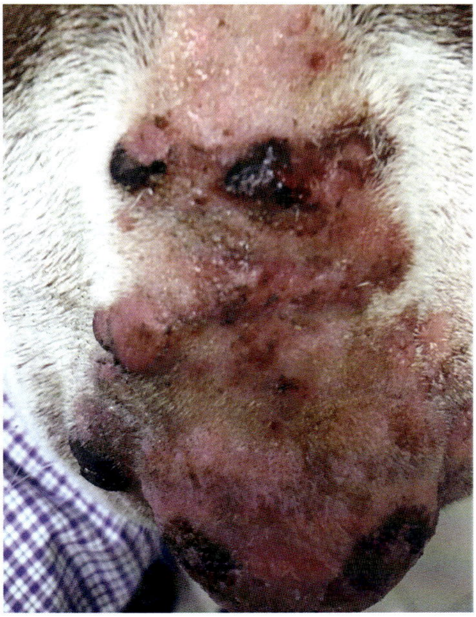

**Figure 16.** Eosinophilic furunculosis and draining tracts.

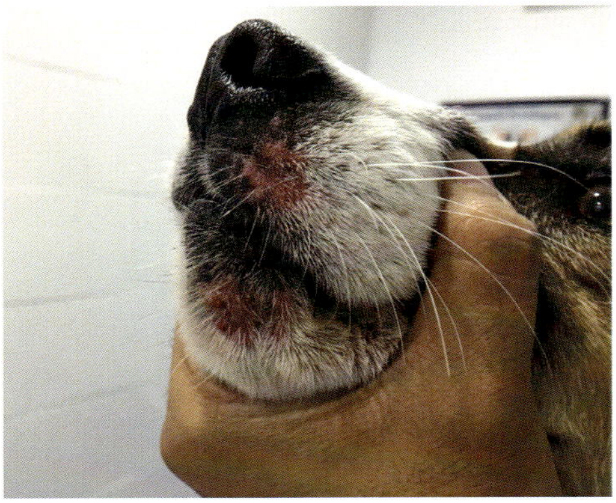

**Figure 17.** Eosinophilic furunculosis on the nasal plane of a dog.

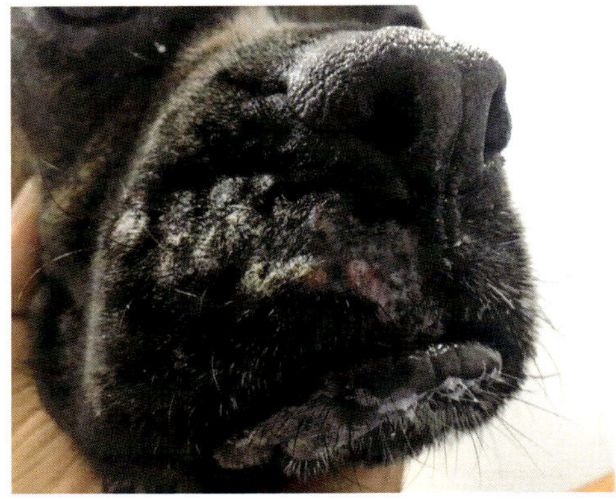

**Figure 18.** Papules and draining tracts in a dog with eosinophilic furunculosis.

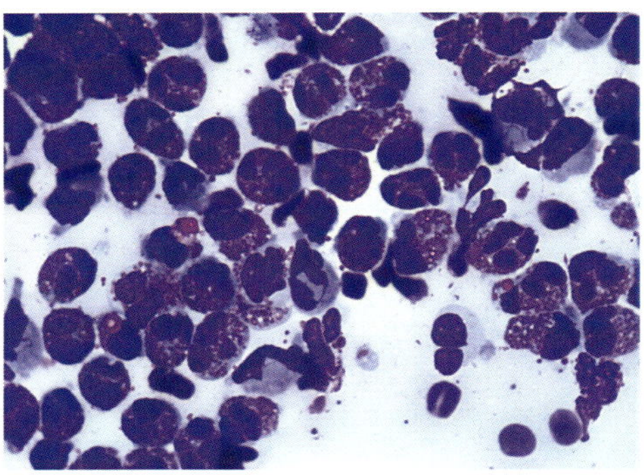

**Figure 19.** Cytology in a case of eosinophilic furunculosis showing an eosinophilic inflammatory reaction with the presence of some macrophages and neutrophils.


## SUMMARY

- Callus pyoderma develops at pressure points, particularly in areas of skin covering bony prominences. Management of this condition requires environmental measures; incidence can be reduced by providing animals with soft mattresses.
- Juvenile pyoderma, or puppy strangles, is a sterile inflammatory disease that affects puppies between 3 weeks and 4 months of age. The treatment of choice is corticosteroids at immunosuppressive doses.
- The first lesions to appear in animals with acne are comedones on the chin and lips. Folliculitis, furunculosis, and suppurative cellulitis may develop in severe cases.
- Facial folliculitis and eosinophilic furunculosis mainly affect the face. Because the cause is an underlying hypersensitivity reaction, patients respond rapidly to corticosteroid treatment.

05

# BACTERIAL CULTURE AND INTERPRETATION OF RESULTS

Bacterial culture is a tool used to identify the type of bacteria present in an infection and subsequently test its sensitivity to antibiotics. Based on the results, the clinician can choose the most appropriate antimicrobial tool for each specific case.

Although sample collection and the interpretation of results are relatively straightforward, specific guidelines should be followed to maximise the clinical efficacy of this diagnostic test.

Before beginning, we must first outline what we expect from the results.

Different sample collection techniques are used for bacterial culture depending on the bacteria involved. In this chapter we will only cover techniques relevant to the collection of samples for skin cultures.

## Choice of laboratory

When selecting a laboratory to perform the bacterial culture it is important to be aware of the available facilities and technologies. Some laboratories offer a range of clinical analyses but do not have the necessary tools or facilities to provide reliable results.

Well-established laboratories are the best option for these types of diagnostic tests. However, most specialise primarily in human medicine. Once the laboratory that will carry out the bacterial culture has been selected, it should be provided with the necessary information on bacterial typing and breakpoints of antibiotics in veterinary medicine in order to ensure optimal results.

## Criteria for sampling for bacterial culture

Bacterial culture is used to identify the causal agent in bacterial infections and subsequently perform antibiotic sensitivity testing, thereby ensuring selection of a viable and effective antimicrobial agent for the patient in question.

A bacterial culture should be requested in the following situations:

- When no clinical response to the initially prescribed antibiotic is observed after 2 weeks of treatment and cytology indicates a persistent infection.
- When bacterial infection persists in patients who have been previously treated with more than 2 different antibiotics over a period of 3 months.

## Cytology in the diagnosis and treatment of bacterial infections

Any treatment for a bacterial infection that includes antibiotic therapy should be based on cytological findings. Without cytology it can be difficult to distinguish between bacterial overgrowth and bacterial infection. Cytology is essential when deciding upon a systemic antibiotic treatment or topical therapy. The latter is effective in most cases of bacterial overgrowth.

Cytology, performed during follow-up examinations, is also one of the best means of assessing the efficacy of antimicrobial therapy. Based on the cytological findings the necessary changes in treatment can be made.

## Recurrence should not be mistaken for resistance

Bacteria can develop mechanisms of resistance that confer immunity to treatment with certain families of antibiotics, inhibiting their action.

Recent years have seen an increase in the population of methicillin-resistant *Staphylococcus pseudintermedius* (MRSP). Through expression of the mecA gene, which encodes penicillin-binding protein 2A (PBP2A), MRSP can avoid the effects of β-lactam antibiotics. MRSP can also display multidrug resistance, i.e. resistance to multiple medications commonly used in the treatment of *S. pseudintermedius.*

MRSP was first reported in North America in 1999 and its prevalence has since increased significantly in European countries and throughout the rest of the world.

**Main factors that have led to the exponential increase in bacterial resistance**

- Prolonged use of antibiotics
- Interruption of antibiotic therapy by clinician or client before resolution of pyoderma
- Use of quinolones for infections that can be resolved using first-choice antibiotics
- Disposal of medications in the rubbish and/or environment
- Repeated use of antibiotics in patients with recurring secondary bacterial infections

It is important that clinicians are able to distinguish between recurrence and bacterial resistance, particularly in cases in which patients develop secondary infections due to an underlying disease, as occurs in allergic patients.

If a given treatment effectively controls an infection, which later reappears, this can be considered a recurrence. By contrast, antibacterial treatment is ineffective in cases of resistance.

## Materials

### Transport medium for bacterial cultures

#### Technique

Samples can be collected from intact pustules or nodules. Intact pustules should be gently cleaned with alcohol and allowed to dry. A 26-gauge needle is used to puncture the pustule and the purulent material within is collected for bacterial culture on the tip of a swab.

In superficial pyoderma patients with no pustules, samples can be obtained from a papule by vigorously rubbing the tip of the swab on the papule.

In patients with epidermal collarettes, samples should be collected from the periphery of the collarettes. The edge of the crust is lifted and the swab rubbed vigorously across the underlying surface (Fig. 1). If the patient does not have epidermal collarettes with a crusted edge, a swab can be rubbed vigorously across the affected area 3 or 4 times (no pre-preparation required) (Figs. 2–5).

In patients with draining tracts, samples should be acquired by inserting the swab into the deepest part of the lesion.

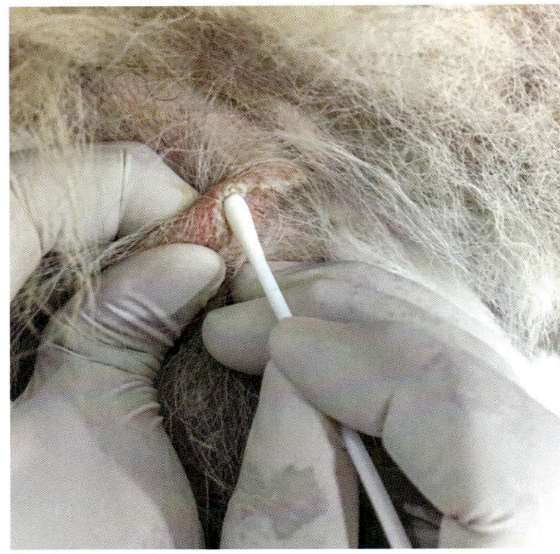

**Figure 1.** Sampling of an epidermal collarette. The sample should be acquired from the edge of the collarette by raising the crust with a swab or sterile needle.

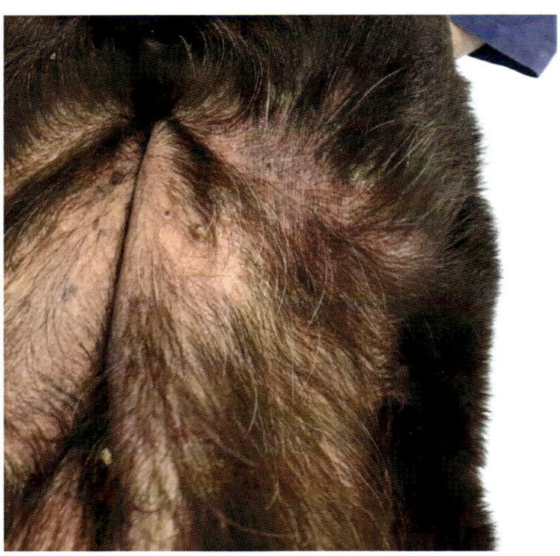

**Figure 2.** Erythematous lesion caused by an epidermal collarette.

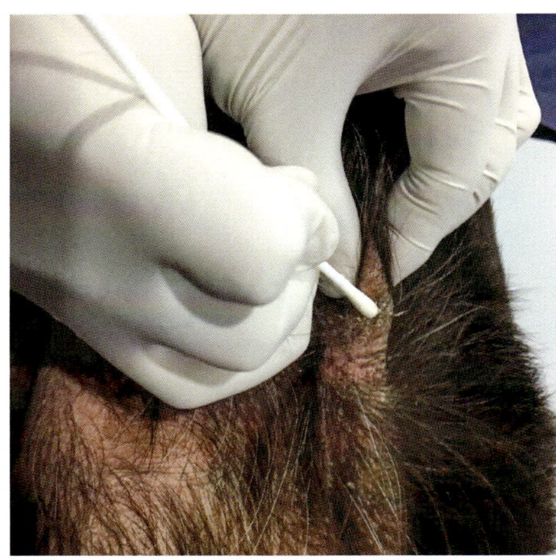

**Figure 3.** In erythematous lesions that have no crust, a sample can be obtained by vigorously rubbing a swab across the affected area.

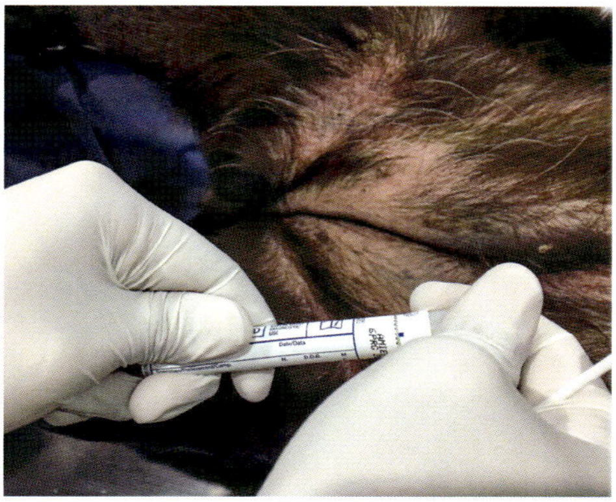

**Figure 4.** The transport medium tube is opened after collecting the sample.

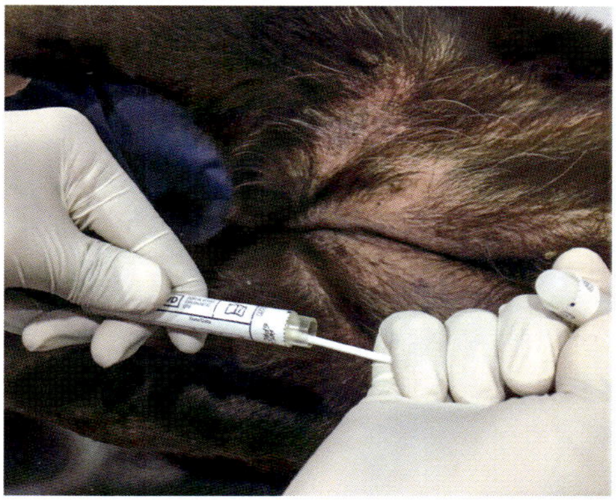

**Figure 5.** The swab bearing the sample is placed into the transport medium (gel) tube for submission to the microbiology laboratory.

**Table 1.** Recommendations for sample collection depending on lesion type.

| Lesion type | Sample collection method |
| --- | --- |
| **Papule** | Vigorously rub the swab across the papule. |
| **Pustule** | Clean the intact pustule with alcohol and puncture with a 26-gauge needle. Collect the exudate with the tip of the swab provided with the transport medium tube. |
| **Epidermal collarette** | Use a swab or sterile needle to raise the crust from the periphery of the lesion and rub vigorously with the swab provided with the transport medium tube. |
| **Epidermal collarette (with no peripheral crust)** | Vigorously rub the swab provided with the transport medium tube across the lesion 3 or 4 times (no prior preparation of the lesion is required). |
| **Draining tracts** | Introduce the swab provided with the transport medium tube deep into the lesion. If necessary, a thinner swab can be used to reach the bottom of the tract. |
| **Crust** | Remove the crust and place it inside the transport medium tube for submission to the laboratory. |
| **Ears** | Insert the swab into the ear at the junction of the vertical and horizontal canals. In cases of stenosis saline solution (0.5 ml) can be introduced via a small-calibre feeding tube to collect the sample by lavage. |
| **Nodule** | To send a nodule to the laboratory to perform a macerated tissue culture, the site of the nodule must first be surgically prepared, after which the nodule is sampled using a 6–8 mm punch and placed in a tube of sterile saline solution without bacteriostatic agents. |

## Minimum inhibitory concentration and breakpoints

**Culture and antimicrobial sensitivity testing are primarily used to identify the causative agent(s) and determine antibiotic susceptibility in order to establish targeted therapy.**

To determine the sensitivity of an agent to an antibiotic, it is necessary to determine its minimum inhibitory concentration (MIC) and the corresponding breakpoint.

The MIC of a causative agent indicates its relative degree of sensitivity to each antibiotic tested. By determining this parameter, the least toxic and most effective medication can be selected.

The purpose of a sensitivity test, regardless of the method used, is to try to match the potency of a drug to a population of pathogens based on the pharmacokinetics of the antimicrobial agent and, where possible, to confirm this relationship through clinical experience and the results of clinical trials.

Breakpoints are discriminatory antimicrobial concentrations used in the interpretation of sensitivity test results to identify isolates as sensitive, intermediate, or resistant. Clinical, pharmacological, microbiological, and pharmacodynamic parameters are considered when establishing breakpoints. The ideal combination of these factors is a topic of continuous debate.

There are official bodies responsible for determining breakpoints through drug diffusion studies and establishing international standards, thereby creating a basis for the determination of bacterial resistance. These include the European Committee Antimicrobial Susceptibility Testing (EUCAST) and the Clinical and Laboratory Standards Institute (CLSI). The main function of in vitro laboratory antimicrobial sensitivity testing is to provide clinicians with information based on which they can select the most appropriate therapy for their patients.

EUCAST has proposed the following definitions for the categorisation of isolates:

1. Clinically resistant: a microorganism is categorised as clinically resistant when its level of antimicrobial sensitivity is greater than expected when the antibiotic is administered systemically. A microorganism is categorised as clinically resistant (R) by applying the appropriate breakpoint in a defined phenotypic test system.

2. Clinically sensitive: a microorganism is defined as clinically sensitive when its level of antimicrobial sensitivity is associated with a high likelihood of therapeutic success. A microorganism is categorised as clinically sensitive (S) by applying the appropriate breakpoint in a defined phenotypic test system.
3. Clinically intermediate: a microorganism is defined as clinically intermediate by a level of antimicrobial activity associated with an uncertain therapeutic effect.

Breakpoints are determined based on the fact that an organism defined as sensitive should respond to the usual dose of a given agent. The rationale for determining the clinical breakpoint is predicated on the fact that an organism designated as susceptible should respond to the usual dose of the agent. A resistant organism should not respond, while one with intermediate susceptibility may or may not respond to the standard dose. In the latter case the organism may respond to a higher dose, provided that there is an active concentration of the antimicrobial agent in the area of the infection. This can pose a problem, as often this information is not available. Furthermore, there are many cases of patients with resistant infections that respond to the medication even though the culture findings suggest the opposite.

## Choice of antimicrobial drug

Selection of the appropriate drug should not be based solely on the results of the bacterial culture and sensitivity test, particularly in the case of skin conditions, since drugs selected based on antibiotic sensitivity test results can often have unwanted adverse effects.

Because the skin is an external organ, topical therapies can be considered as potential treatment options for bacterial infections.

Antibiotic sensitivity profiles can suggest therapeutic options such as aminoglycosides or other medications that have a high nephrotoxic potential, and may even promote resistance. As clinical veterinary surgeons, we should resist the temptation to prescribe these medications and instead rely on topical therapy with shampoos and solutions (as discussed in depth in the next chapter).

However, in cases in which there are viable options available that do not generate unnecessary risks for the patient, the MIC can be used to select the antimicrobial drug that best suits the patient. The drug selected should be that with an MIC as far away as possible from values corresponding to intermediate sensitivity. If viable options are of intermediate sensitivity, the highest permitted dose of the drug should be selected in order to increase the drug's concentration at the affected site.

It is important to collect data on bacterial resistance in different geographical areas in order to facilitate more accurate and global evaluation of bacterial resistance.

## SUMMARY

- Bacterial culture should be requested in cases in which the chosen therapy does not provide a positive outcome, either clinically or cytologically.
- Bacterial culture can be used in patients who have not responded to treatment with several antimicrobial agents administered discontinuously or over a short period of time.
- The choice of antimicrobial medication should not be based solely on the results of the culture and sensitivity testing.
- The toxic potential of candidate drugs should always be taken into account, as well as the dose required to achieve therapeutic concentrations.
- Knowledge of the mechanism of action of each drug and the appropriate concentration for the treatment of skin conditions is key to selecting the appropriate treatment.

06

# TOPICAL TREATMENT OF BACTERIAL SKIN INFECTIONS

Topical treatment is the therapeutic application of a medication externally and locally using a variety of vehicles, such as shampoos, gels, creams, ointments, lotions, sprays, and drops. Topical treatment has always been a fundamental component of the therapeutic management of dermatological problems.

Before the development of systemic therapies, topical treatment was used to sooth, disinfect, moisturise, or dry the skin of patients, both animal and human, with dermatological problems.

This chapter will discuss a variety of agents with antimicrobial properties that have shown beneficial effects in the treatment of bacterial infections of dogs and cats.

The increase in bacterial resistance observed in recent years constitutes a latent risk to future generations, and has obliged health professionals to adopt a more specific therapeutic approach. Only a few years ago the range of available active substances for topical use was quite limited. However, nowadays there is a wide range of options that are both user-friendly in terms of formulation and aroma and have a high degree of antimicrobial efficacy.

## General principles of topical therapy

Multiple agents are used for the treatment of bacterial skin infections. These agents are available in different formulations depending on:

- Site of application
- Mechanism of action and the distribution of the active substance
- Combination with other pharmacological agents (anti-inflammatories, anti-fungals, anaesthetics)
- Frequency of application by the owner

The following vehicles are used for the delivery of active ingredients for the treatment of bacterial skin infections in dogs and cats:

- Shampoos
- Creams
- Gels
- Ointments
- Impregnated wipes
- Sprays
- Lotions
- Ointments

## Antimicrobial agents and their mechanisms of action

As mentioned above, multiple antimicrobial agents with different mechanisms of action are used to treat bacterial skin infections. It is important that veterinary clinicians are able to choose the most appropriate antimicrobial agent for each situation and that this decision is based not only on clinical signs, but also on the results of cytological and microbiological analyses and the type of patient.

### Chlorhexidine

Chlorhexidine is considered an antimicrobial agent and is used at concentrations of 0.5–4 %. Its mode of action consists of eliminating bacteria by inducing the coagulation of cytoplasmic proteins, resulting in deterioration of the cell wall.

Several studies evaluating the appropriate concentration of chlorhexidine for antibacterial purposes have proposed concentrations ranging from 2 % to 4 %. Another study comparing the effectiveness of 4 % chlorhexidine shampoo with systemic therapy with amoxicillin and clavulanic acid demonstrated the effectiveness of shampoo for the treatment of methicillin-susceptible and methicillin-resistant pyoderma.

The combination of chlorhexidine and miconazole may exert a synergistic antibacterial effect.

### Miconazole

Although miconazole is considered an antifungal agent, some studies have described synergistic effects when combined with chlorhexidine. This combination can be very useful for the treatment of allergic patients, in which secondary bacterial and yeast infections are common.

Miconazole is effective against yeasts. *Malassezia* spp. are the most common yeast species in inflammatory skin conditions. *Malassezia* can be a complicating factor in allergic patients and some patients may become sensitised, resulting in an exacerbated allergic response in the presence of these yeasts.

## Benzoyl peroxide

Benzoyl peroxide is commonly used at concentrations of 2.5 % to 3 %. It is an oxidizing agent and its mode of action consists of damaging the bacterial cell wall, thereby increasing permeability and ultimately causing cell rupture.

Upon contact with the skin benzoyl peroxide decomposes to benzoic acid and oxygen. The generation of highly reactive oxygen radicals results in oxidation of bacteria, a physico-chemical effect not associated with bacterial resistance. Benzoic acid is responsible for the inhibition of epidermal proliferation and sebum production. The decrease in free fatty acids in sebum may be due to the antibacterial effect associated with the inhibition of bacterial lipases.

Frequent use can result in irritation and/or dryness in some patients.

Benzoyl peroxide has a follicular cleansing action, and therefore is used preferentially for deep infections in which folliculitis and furunculosis are present. It also exerts keratolytic, comedolytic, anti-inflammatory, and bleaching effects, making it useful for seborrhoeic infectious processes.

It has no antifungal effects.

## Ethyl lactate

Ethyl lactate is metabolised to ethanol and lactic acid by bacterial lipases in hair follicles and sebaceous glands. Ethanol solubilises lipids and lactic acid decreases the skin's pH, resulting in a bactericidal effect.

Its effect is facilitated by its ability to spread through the different layers of the skin.

## Tin fluoride

Tin combined with fluoride has been used in human dental hygiene since it was first shown to cause a marked decrease in bacterial counts in saliva samples. This decrease was attributed to the antibacterial action of tin ions.

It is used most commonly in horses as a 0.4 % gel to treat dermatophilosis and staphylococcal infections. A study in dogs demonstrated its effectiveness in the treatment of pyoderma when administered as a 0.2 % spray, although no significant difference was observed with respect to the placebo group. Therefore, it is not recommended for the treatment of bacterial skin infections in dogs.

## Triclosan

Triclosan belongs to the family of bisphenols and exerts antibacterial activity against gram-positive bacteria. Gram-negative bacteria, particularly *Pseudomonas aeruginosa,* are more resistant to this compound. Its mechanism of action is not fully characterised. Triclosan resistance has been reported in strains of methicillin-resistant *Staphylococcus.*

It is found in antibacterial soap and shampoos. However, more studies are required to better evaluate its effectiveness in dogs.

## Mupirocin

In some countries mupirocin is approved for the treatment of pyoderma in dogs. It is sold as a 2 % ointment and is reportedly effective for the treatment of certain strains of resistant staphylococci in humans. It is used frequently to treat feline acne and exerts a strong antibacterial effect.

## Silver compounds

Silver ions exert an antibacterial effect by interacting with certain groups of proteins and bacterial enzymes, inhibiting cell division of nucleic acids and damaging their cell walls.

Silver sulfadiazine binds bacterial DNA and inhibits its transcription. Some products combine silver sulfadiazine with a quinolone to enhance this antibacterial effect.

Certain compounds contain silver nanoparticles (approximately 10 μm) that continuously produce ions in the skin. These remain on the skin surface and eliminate bacteria. These compounds are formed by the exposure of medicinal-grade 99.97 % silver to high temperatures.

## Phytosphingosine

This is a sphingosine derived from plants, and consists of an amino acid and a fatty acid. It exerts antifungal effects, by blocking amino acid synthesis, and antibacterial effects at concentrations of over 0.04 %.

In addition to its antimicrobial effect, it inhibits protein kinase C and plays an important role in the regulation of cell growth. It can also inhibit interleukin-1 (IL-1) in skin exposed to UVB rays.

## Povidone iodine

Iodine exerts a rapid antibacterial effect by penetrating cells and damaging fatty acids, nucleotides, and intracellular proteins, causing cell death. It exerts bactericidal, fungicidal, virucidal, and sporocidal effects.

Aqueous solutions prepared with povidone iodine are usually unstable. Its effect in veterinary medicine has been compared with that of chlorhexidine, although povidone iodine causes more marked skin irritation in up to 50 % of cases.

## Sodium hypochlorite

Chlorine or sodium hypochlorite has a broad bactericidal, virucidal, fungicidal, and sporocidal effect.

Some studies have evaluated the antibacterial effects of chlorine and its potential as a therapeutic agent in infections caused by methicillin-resistant as well as methicillin-susceptible *Staphylococcus* species. One study demonstrated that in addition to its antibacterial effect, sodium hypochlorite can reduce the induction of inflammatory genes in keratinocytes without causing alterations in skin lipids and ceramides. It causes no skin irritation at concentrations of 0.05–0.005 %.

Sodium hypochlorite is an excellent option for the treatment of resistant pyoderma.

### SUMMARY

- The choice of topical therapy depends on the clinical presentation of the infection, the cytological findings, and the owner's ability to administer the treatment.
- Different vehicles are used to deliver the active substances. The choice of vehicle will depend on the extent and severity of the lesion, the patient, and the type of active substance.
- Topical therapy (Table 1) should complement or even replace systemic treatment whenever possible to reduce the likelihood that bacterial resistance develops.

**Table 1.** Main characteristics of the active ingredients most commonly used for topical antibacterial treatment.

| Active substance | Main effects | Formulation |
|---|---|---|
| **Chlorhexidine 2–4 %** | Eliminates bacteria by inducing protein coagulation in the cytoplasm and damaging the cell wall. | ■ Shampoo<br>■ Solution<br>■ Impregnated wipe |
| **Benzoyl peroxide 2.5–3.0 %** | ■ Increases permeability of the bacterial cell wall, causing its rupture.<br>■ Comedolytic.<br>■ Keratolytic. | ■ Shampoo<br>■ Gel<br>■ Ointment |
| **Miconazole/clotrimazole** | ■ Antifungal agent.<br>■ Antibacterial when combined with chlorhexidine (enhanced effect). | ■ Shampoo<br>■ Solution<br>■ Impregnated wipe |
| **Ethyl lactate** | Ethanol solubilises lipids and lactic acid decreases the skin's pH, producing a bactericidal effect. | ■ Shampoo |
| **Tin fluoride 0.2–0.4 %** | ■ Tin ions exert antibacterial action.<br>■ Efficacy in canine pyoderma not demonstrated. | ■ Solution<br>■ Gel |
| **Triclosan** | Antibacterial activity against gram-positive bacteria. | ■ Soap<br>■ Shampoo<br>■ Solution |
| **Mupirocin 2 %** | ■ Antibacterial effect (including resistant strains).<br>■ Feline acne.<br>■ Canine pyoderma. | ■ Ointment |
| **Silver compounds** | Antibacterial effect owing to its interaction with certain groups of proteins and bacterial enzymes. | ■ Shampoo<br>■ Solution<br>■ Ointment |
| **Phytosphingosine 0.04 %** | ■ Antifungal action caused by the blockade of amino acid synthesis.<br>■ Antibacterial effect. | ■ Solution |
| **Povidone iodine** | ■ Bactericidal, virucidal, fungicidal, sporocidal effects.<br>■ Irritation in 50 % of cases. | ■ Solution |
| **Sodium hypochlorite 0.005–0.05 %** | Bactericidal, virucidal, fungicidal, sporocidal effect. | ■ Solution |

07

# SYSTEMIC TREATMENT OF BACTERIAL SKIN INFECTIONS

Systemic antibiotics are a fundamental tool for the treatment of bacterial skin infections. However, the use of these types of therapies has decreased in recent years with the increasing incidence of bacterial resistance.

As discussed in other chapters, the choice of treatment is based on cytological findings, clinical signs, the type of patient, and the owner's ability to administer the treatment. The systemic antibiotics most commonly used in veterinary dermatology belong to the penicillin, sulfonamide, macrolide, lincosamide, cephalosporin, and fluoroquinolone families. Antibiotics used to treat skin conditions must have a narrow spectrum in order to minimise their effects on the cutaneous and intestinal microbiota. Antibiotics with bactericidal effects are preferable, although certain bacteriostatic agents can also be used provided that the patient is not immunocompromised.

**Two key considerations when administering systemic antibiotics to treat bacterial skin infections are bacterial susceptibility and the distribution of the drug through the skin.**

Regarding drug distribution in the skin, it should be borne in mind that the skin accounts for 4 % of cardiac output, as compared with 33 % in the case of muscle. For this reason, it is important to adhere to the recommended dose range for each product. However, in the case of more severe infections higher doses can be used, always respecting the recommended dose intervals and duration of treatment.

**Factors that can decrease the effectiveness of systemic treatment of bacterial skin infections**

- Sensitivity of the infectious agent.
- Doses that are inadequate to ensure appropriate concentrations in the skin.
- Presence of scar tissue, which can prevent the spread of the antibiotic to the site of infection.
- Presence of a foreign body, such as hair particles, in a necrotic centre in a skin lesion.
- Inadequate duration of antibiotic treatment.
- Survival of organisms within macrophages.

## Selection of systemic antibiotics

Ideally, selection of a systemic antibiotic for the treatment of a given patient should be based on the results of bacterial culture and sensitivity testing. However, this is impractical in daily practice owing to the cost and time required to perform a culture for each patient with a bacterial skin infection. Therefore, as mentioned above, the selection of an antibiotic should be based on cytological findings and clinical signs.

Another key factor when choosing an antibiotic is to limit the selection to those that have a narrow spectrum but are effective against *Staphylococcus pseudintermedius* and other coccoid bacteria identified by cytology.

In recent years, with the emergence of other families of broad-spectrum antibiotics such as quinolones, many veterinary professionals have started to prescribe these agents in a more general manner for the treatment of a wide range of infections (urinary, cutaneous, respiratory, digestive, etc.). The excessive use of these molecules led to an increase in bacterial resistance, against which an important battle is currently being waged.

It is advisable to be conservative when prescribing systemic treatments for pyoderma and to resist the temptation to use broad-spectrum and last-generation antibiotics. These should be reserved for the most difficult cases, or those in which their use is justified based on the results of sensitivity testing.

## Treatment duration

The duration of treatment will depend on the severity and depth of the infection. In general, superficial pyoderma requires 2 to 3 weeks of treatment, and as a rule treatment should be continued for 1 to 2 weeks after clinical resolution. Therefore deep pyoderma, which requires 2 to 4 weeks to resolve, will require a total treatment duration of 4 to 6 weeks.

Clinical findings must be considered when determining when to finish treatment: lesions should be palpated and a decrease in their extent should be evident. If the problem recurs between 2 and 21 days after completing treatment it is likely that the infection had not resolved and required more prolonged treatment.

Another factor that should be taken into account is that the concurrent administration of corticosteroids alongside antibiotics can help reduce follicular inflammation, but can also create the impression of improvement, leading clinicians to end systemic treatment earlier than necessary and thereby perpetuating the infection.

## Owner compliance

One of the biggest problems encountered in the treatment of bacterial skin infections is owner compliance with treatment guidelines.

**Factors that may favour owner compliance**

- Prescription of medicines that require once-daily administration
- Use of palatable or easy-to-administer tablets
- Effective communication with the owner
- Detailed instructions accompanying the prescription
- Administration of long-acting injectable drugs
- Dispensing of the exact amount of drug required
- Use of smartphones applications to provide reminders

If no clinical improvement is observed after the first 2 weeks of treatment, assuming that the antibiotic was selected based on clinical and cytological findings, a culture and antibiotic sensitivity test are highly recommended.

**Table 1.** Recommendations for the use of antimicrobial agents for superficial bacterial folliculitis, based on published literature (Hillier et al., 2014).

| Class of antimicrobial agent | When to use it | Antimicrobial drug |
|---|---|---|
| **First choice** | First choice for empirical treatment of superficial and deep bacterial infections. | ■ Clindamycin<br>■ Lincomycin<br>■ Enhanced sulfonamide<br>■ Cephalexin<br>■ Amoxicillin–clavulanic acid |
| **Second choice** | When the first choice is considered inappropriate based on bacterial culture and sensitivity testing. | ■ Doxycycline<br>■ Chloramphenicol<br>■ Fluroquinolones<br>■ Rifampicin<br>■ Aminoglycosides (nephrotoxic) |
| **Third option** | When the first and second choices are considered inappropriate based on bacterial culture and sensitivity testing | ■ Linezolid<br>■ Teicoplanin<br>■ Vancomycin (restricted use) |

**Table 2.** Systemic antimicrobial agents most commonly used for bacterial skin infections: doses and adverse effects.

| Antimicrobial agent | Dose | Adverse effects |
|---|---|---|
| **Narrow spectrum** | | |
| **Erythromycin** | 15 mg/kg every 8 h or 15–25 mg/kg every 12 hours | ■ Common: vomiting<br>■ Rare: nausea, anorexia, diarrhoea, abdominal pain, liver dysfunction and elevated liver enzyme levels, allergic reactions (urticaria, mild skin rashes, anaphylaxis) |
| **Clindamycin** | 11 mg/kg every 12–24 h | ■ Common: vomiting, diarrhoea, anorexia.<br>■ Rare: bloody diarrhoea, esophagitis, oesophageal constriction in cats when not administered with water, cutaneous allergic reaction, neuromuscular blockade, leukopenia, elevated liver enzyme levels |
| **Lincomycin** | 22 mg/12 h | - |
| **Tylosin** | 10–20 mg/kg every 12 h | - |
| **Broad spectrum** | | |
| **Azithromycin** | 5–10 mg/kg every 12–24 h | ■ Common: vomiting, diarrhoea, anorexia, abdominal pain.<br>■ Rare: hepatomegaly, cholestatic hepatitis, elevated liver enzyme levels, phospholipidosis |

▶

| Antimicrobial agent | Dose | Adverse effects |
|---|---|---|
| **Amoxicillin–clavulanic acid** | 12.5–25 mg/kg every 12 h | ■ Common: vomiting, diarrhoea, anorexia<br>■ Rare: adverse skin reactions, lethargy, depression, polyuria, polydipsia, claudication, behavioural changes, tachypnoea, neurotoxicity, elevation of liver enzymes, dyspnoea, tachycardia |
| **Cephalexin** | 30 mg/12 h | ■ Common: vomiting, diarrhoea, anorexia<br>■ Rare: salivation, tachypnoea, excitability, lethargy, hypersensitivity reactions, urticaria, nephrotoxicity, erythema multiforme, drug-induced pemphigus, transient increases in liver enzyme levels |
| **Cefpodoxime** | 5–10 mg/kg every 24 h | ■ Common: vomiting, diarrhoea, anorexia<br>■ Rare: lethargy, hypersensitivity reactions, nephrotoxicity, coagulation disorders |
| **Cefovecin** | 8 mg/kg SC every 14 days | ■ Common: vomiting, soft stools, diarrhoea, decreased appetite, anorexia, lethargy, mild injection site reactions (inflammation or pruritus)<br>■ Rare: bloody stools, flatulence, elevated liver enzyme levels, injection site reactions (seroma, alopecia, crusting, necrosis, erythema), facial oedema, tremors, acute pulmonary oedema, excessive salivation, pruritus, haemolytic anaemia, ataxia, seizures |
| **Cefadroxil** | 22–30 mg/kg every 12 h | ■ Common: anorexia, vomiting, diarrhoea, lethargy (administration with food is recommended)<br>■ Rare: cutaneous hypersensitivity reactions, fever, eosinophilia, lymphadenopathy, anaphylaxis |
| **Chloramphenicol** | 40–60 mg/kg every 8 h | ■ Common: vomiting, diarrhoea, anorexia, depression<br>■ Rare: exercise intolerance, weakness, tachycardia, weight loss, bone marrow suppression (high doses or prolonged treatment, reversible with cessation of treatment) |
| **Clarithromycin** | 5–10 mg/kg every 12 h | ■ Common: diarrhoea, vomiting, nausea, anorexia<br>■ Rare: erythema of the ears, orange coloration of the skin |
| **Difloxacin** | 5–10 mg/kg every 24 h | ■ Common: nausea, vomiting, diarrhoea, anorexia, arthropathy in young animals<br>■ Rare: central nervous system toxicity (high doses), especially in patients with renal failure |
| **Enrofloxacin** | 5–20 mg/kg every 24 h | ■ Common: vomiting, diarrhoea, anorexia, elevated liver enzyme levels<br>■ Rare: cartilage abnormalities in young animals, ataxia, seizures, depression, lethargy, aggression, vocalisation, anxiety |
| **Marbofloxacin** | 2.5–5 mg/kg every 24 h | Well tolerated in general but can cause nausea, vomiting, diarrhoea, soft stools, lethargy, seizures (high doses) |

| Antimicrobial agent | Dose | Adverse effects |
|---|---|---|
| **Orbifloxacin** | 2.5–7.5 mg/kg every 24 h | Well tolerated in general but can cause nausea, vomiting, diarrhoea, soft stools, lethargy |
| **Pradofloxacin** | 3–4.5 mg/kg every 24 h | Well tolerated in general but can cause nausea, vomiting, diarrhoea, soft stools, lethargy |
| **Trimethoprim sulfa** | 30 mg/kg every 24 h or 15 mg/kg every 12 h | Fever, thrombocytopaenia, hepatopathy, keratoconjunctivitis sicca, neutropaenia, haemolytic anaemia, crystalluria, arthropathy, uveitis, cutaneous and mucocutaneous lesions, urticaria, angioedema, proteinuria, facial paralysis, clinical signs of hypothyroidism (high doses and prolonged treatment), diarrhoea, vomiting, anorexia, seizures |
| **Miscellaneous** | | |
| **Doxycycline** | 5–10 mg/kg every 12–24 h | ■ Common: nausea, vomiting, diarrhoea, anorexia (administration with food is recommended)<br>■ Rare: oesophageal constriction (cats), growth of nonsusceptible bacteria or fungi, photosensitivity reactions, hepatotoxicity, blood dyscrasia |
| **Rifampicin** | 5–10 mg/kg every 12–24 h | Hepatotoxicity (high doses and prolonged treatment), pancreatitis, thrombocytopaenia, haemolytic anaemia, anorexia, vomiting, diarrhoea, death, reddish colouration of urine, saliva, and tears |
| **Aminoglycosides (injectable, not recommended in cases of nephrotoxicity)** | | |
| **Tobramycin** | 9–14 mg/kg SC every 24 h | Nephrotoxicity, ototoxicity |
| **Netilmicin** | 9–14 mg/kg SC every 24 h | Nephrotoxicity, ototoxicity |
| **Amikacin** | 15–30 mg/kg SC every 24 h | Nephrotoxicity, ototoxicity |
| **Gentamicin** | 9–14 mg/kg SC every 24 h | Nephrotoxicity, ototoxicity |

## SUMMARY

- Antibiotics used to treat skin conditions must have a narrow spectrum and bactericidal action.
- In practice, the best way to choose an antibiotic is to base the selection on cytological findings and clinical signs.
- The duration of treatment depends on the severity and depth of the infection.
- Owner compliance with treatment guidelines is essential to ensure success.

08

# MECHANISMS OF BACTERIAL RESISTANCE

Since the introduction of antibiotics, bacteria have been engaged in a fight for their survival and have evolved mechanisms to ensure their permanence in the face of changes in both their internal and external environment.

**The excessive use and unnecessary prescription of antibiotics and repeated treatments without prescription are some of the factors that have favoured the development of bacterial resistance mechanisms.**

In the case of veterinary dermatology, a key driver of bacterial resistance is the failure to control or treat the underlying causes of bacterial skin infections, which consequently recur. As discussed in the preceding chapters, patients with skin conditions often develop secondary bacterial infections caused by a range of different factors, including allergies and immunosuppression. Consequently, some patients with these chronic conditions can develop numerous secondary bacterial infections throughout the course of their lives. In many cases this situation leads to repeated antibiotic treatment, which in turn can give rise to bacterial resistance.

## Methicillin-resistant *Staphylococcus pseudintermedius* (MRSP)

*Staphylococcus pseudintermedius* is one of the main agents implicated in canine pyoderma and one of the bacteria most commonly mentioned in the context of antibiotic-resistant skin bacteria. MRSP (methicillin-resistant *Staphylococcus pseudintermedius*) was first described in North America in 1999. In the early days of bacterial resistance, *Staphylococcus aureus* was identified in human antibiotic-resistant nosocomial infections before discovery of its canine counterpart.

Both displayed resistance to methicillin, an antibiotic used as an indicator of susceptibility to β-lactam antibiotics.

Nowadays, oxacillin is used in antibiotic sensitivity tests instead of methicillin, but the term "methicillin-resistant" is still used to describe oxacillin-resistant organisms.

Recent years have seen an increase in the prevalence of methicillin-resistant bacterial infections in both humans and animals, exceeding 55 % in collected cultures. In most cases MRSP is characterised by expression of the *mecA* gene, which encodes penicillin-binding protein 2a (PBP2a). This altered protein confers resistance to β-lactams, including penicillins, cephalosporins, and carbapenems. In some cases MRSP can present multiresistance to other families of antibiotics, including aminoglycosides, quinolones, tetracyclines, and macrolides. Antibiotic treatment is the only risk factor for the development of MRSP identified to date.

Multiresistance to antibiotics, which is more common in MRSP than MRSA isolates, is one of the greatest concerns in veterinary medicine. A study of 103 isolates collected in North America and Europe found that 90 % of MRSP isolates showed resistance to ciprofloxacin, clindamycin, erythromycin, kanamycin, streptomycin, and trimethoprim. Resistance to gentamicin and tetracycline was observed in 70 % of cases and chloramphenicol resistance in 57 % of cases. Analysis of 72 isolates collected throughout Germany revealed the highest resistance indices, with resistance to quinolones, aminoglycosides, and macrolides detected in up to 97.8 % of cases.

Despite variations in the findings reported in different studies conducted globally, one common element is an increase in the resistance index in recent years. Moreover, many countries in which there was a lack of awareness and information on antibiotic resistance have begun to report cases and generate awareness about the rational use of antibiotics.

## Zoonotic implications of MRSP

Studies of bacterial adherence and colonisation have shown that dogs are colonised primarily by *S. pseudintermedius*, and humans primarily by *S. aureus* and *Staphylococcus epidermidis*. The zoonotic potential of MRSP is nonetheless real, although most reported human cases involve spontaneous colonisation. Cases of owners with deep pyoderma caused by *S. pseudintermedius* strains identical to those of their pets have been reported.

With the emergence of MRSP in animals there has been an increase in studies investigating colonisation by this bacterium of humans who live with animals. Studies of nasal cultures from veterinary personnel revealed that 3–5.3 % of those studied were positive for MRSP.

Similar studies of owners of pets with MRSP infections found that 4–13 % were positive. Moreover, results of genetic analyses of the isolates supported interspecies transmission.

A more recent study found that 8 % of veterinary personnel sampled in a hospital were positive for MRSA, although this was not shared with patients or their pets; 7 % of dogs belonging to patients at the hospital and 8 % of dogs belonging to the tested veterinary surgeons were positive for MRSP. Differences in MRSP clonality were observed between patients and the dogs of veterinary surgeons. MRSP was not detected in any of the veterinary personnel who participated in this study.

It thus appears that MRSP colonisation in humans is rare. Although more studies are needed, it is possible that humans carry MRSP more often than MSSP (methicillin-susceptible *S. pseudintermedius*). This could reflect the occupational risk of MRSA in veterinary personnel and the increased risk to owners with pets with MRSA infections.

## MRSP clonality and variants

Distinct clones of MRSP have been identified in different geographic regions. A systematic review of several studies found that MRSP accounted for 76 % of 1,428 isolates that were characterised by multilocus sequence typing. This population is very diverse and includes the five main clonal complexes (CCs). CC71, previously known as the European clone, is now distributed worldwide. CC258, which is the most susceptible to enrofloxacin and aminoglycosides, and is more frequently resistant to sulfonamides/trimethoprim than CC71, is reported with increasing frequency in various European countries. CC68, previously known as the North American clone, is frequently reported in North America as well as Europe, while CC112 and CC45, which is associated with chloramphenicol resistance, are prevalent in Asia.

Knowledge of existing MRSP clones and their resistance to antibiotics is essential given their increasing prevalence and global distribution. It is therefore necessary to collect data in other countries in order to help characterise the associated epidemiology.

## Biofilm

Bacterial biofilm consists of layers of cell clusters grouped in an extracellular matrix composed of polysaccharides that adhere to inert surfaces. It serves as a protective mechanism by promoting vertical growth of bacteria and the subsequent formation of a protective layer, which in turn allows the bacteria to continue their vertical growth and to spread further.

The ability to form a biofilm has been described in many microorganisms, including *S. pseudintermedius*, although in this species the process is yet to be fully characterised. One study found that the majority (96 %) of *S. pseudintermedius* isolates are capable of producing a moderate or strong biofilm. The strain corresponding to ST-71, the most prevalent sequence type in Europe, has a marked capacity to form a biofilm.

**Stages of biofilm formation**

- Initial reversible adherence of free microorganisms to the surface
- Permanent chemical binding, single layer
- Early vertical development
- Multiple towers with intermediate channels, biofilm maturation
- Mature biofilm with seed production and dispersion of microorganisms

Some studies have shown that the bacteria that grow inside the biofilm are generally more resistant to antibiotics. In addition to antibiotic resistance mechanisms, this resistance may be due to the decrease in the rate of bacterial growth within the mature biofilm and the induction of a biofilm phenotype characterised by the presence of activated multidrug efflux pumps.

**Efflux pumps**

These are mechanisms that allow the direct expulsion of several drugs from the cytosol or periplasmic space to the outside of the bacterial wall, favouring resistance.

## Contamination and disinfection of hospital areas and medical personnel

**Control of MRSP is not exclusively based on the responsible use of antibiotics.**

With the identification of potential reservoirs of drug-resistant staphylococci, greater attention is now being paid to the cleaning and disinfection of hospital areas and medical staff in veterinary hospitals.

It is essential to carefully manage hygiene in consultation areas in clinics and hospitals, and to ensure that personnel clean their hands and disinfect their clothes when dealing with patients with MRSP infection. Clothing is also a potential source of contamination.

In addition to furniture, clothing, and hospital facilities, devices such as mobile phones pose additional risks of contamination. One study in which samples were taken from the telephones of medical personnel confirmed the presence of MRSP and MRSA in 1.6 % (2 of 123) and 0.8 % (1 of 123) of cases, respectively, despite the fact that 21.9 % of the participants reported that they routinely cleaned their phones.

Most cleaning fluids and disinfectants used in hospitals are adequate for routine disinfection. However, chlorine remains a highly effective and economical disinfectant. It is advisable to disinfect more thoroughly after attending to patients with MRSP.

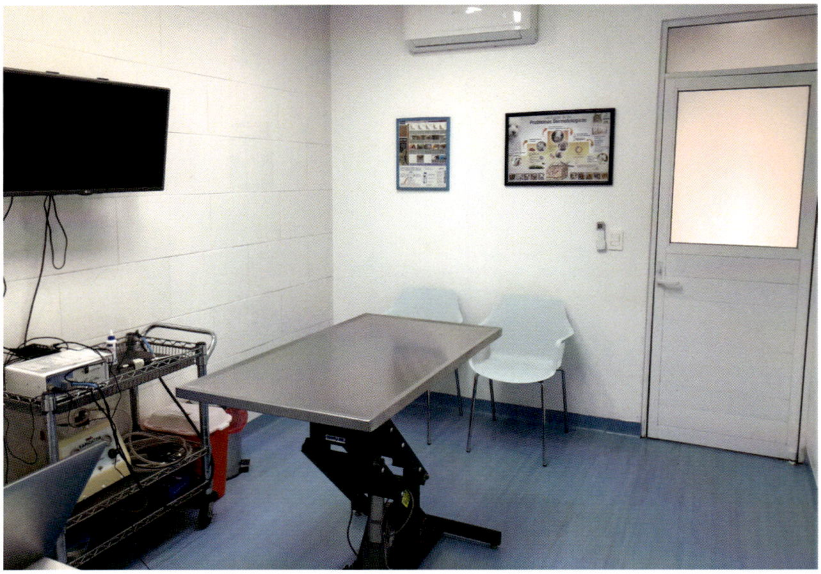

**Figure 1.** Adequate disinfection of the entire consultation area is essential.

## SUMMARY

- The excessive use and unnecessary prescription of antibiotics and repeated treatments without prescription are some of the factors that have favoured the development of bacterial resistance mechanisms.
- *Staphylococcus pseudintermedius* is one of the main agents implicated in canine pyoderma and one of the bacterial species most commonly mentioned in the context of antibiotic-resistant bacterial skin infections.
- Some studies have shown that the bacteria that grow inside the biofilm are generally more resistant to antibiotics.
- The cleaning and disinfection of hospital areas and medical personnel in veterinary hospitals is essential to avoid contamination.

# BIBLIOGRAPHY

## Chapter 1


COHEN, M., BOHLING M.W., WRIGHT J.C., et al. Evaluation of sensitivity and specificity of cytologic examination: 269 cases (1999–2000). *J Am Vet Med Assoc*, 2003; 222(7):964–967.

HUMAN MICROBIOME PROJECT CONSORTIUM. Structure, function and diversity of the healthy human microbiome. *Nature*, 2012; 486:207–214.

INTEGRATIVE HMP (iHMP) RESEARCH NETWORK CONSORTIUM. The Integrative Human Microbiome Project: dynamic analysis of microbiome-host omics profiles during periods of human health and disease. *Cell Host Microbe*, 2014; 16:276–289.

LEDERBERG, J. Infectious history. *Science*, 2000; 288:287–293.

LO, K. L., ROSENKRANTZ, W. S. Evaluation of cytology collection techniques and prevalence of *Malassezia* yeast and bacteria in claw folds of normal and allergic dogs. *Vet Dermatol*, 2016; 27(4):279–e67.

MEASON-SMITH, C., DIESEL, A., PATTERSON, A.P. et al. Characterization of the cutaneous mycobiota in healthy and allergic cats using next-generation sequencing. *Vet Dermatol*, 2016.

MILLER, W. H., GRIFFIN, C. E., CAMPBELL, K. L. *Muller and Kirk's Small Animal Dermatology*, 7th ed, 2013. Elsevier Health Sciences.

NELSON, J. D. Impression cytology. *Cornea*, 1988; 7(1):71–81.

PROCTOR, L. M. The Human Microbiome Project in 2011 and beyond. *Cell Host Microbe*, 2011; 10:287–291.

RANJAN, R., RANI, A., METWALLY, A. et al. Analysis of the microbiome: advantages of whole genome shotgun versus 16S amplicon sequencing. *Biochem Biophys Res Commun*, 2016; 469:967–977.

RODRIGUES HOFFMANN, A., PATTERSON, A.P., DIESEL, A. et al. The skin microbiome in healthy and allergic dogs. *PLoS One*, 2014; 9:e83197.

RODRIGUES HOFFMANN, A. The cutaneous ecosystem: the roles of the skin microbiome in health and its association with inflammatory skin conditions in humans and animals. *Vet Dermatol*, 2017; 28(1):60.

SCHARSCHMIDT, T.C., VASQUEZ, K.S., TRUONG, H.A. et al. A wave of regulatory T cells into neonatal skin mediates tolerance to commensal microbes. *Immunity*, 2015; 43:1011–1021.


## Chapter 2


BAEUMER, W., BIZIKOVA, P., JACOB, M., LINDER, K. E. Establishing a canine superficial pyoderma model. *J Appl Microbiol*, 2017; 122(2):331–337.

BANOVIC, F., LINDER, K., OLIVRY, T. Clinical, microscopic and microbial characterization of exfoliative superficial pyoderma-associated epidermal collarettes in dogs. *Vet Dermatol*, 2017; 28(1):107.

CORDERO, A. M., SHEINBERG-WAISBURD, G., ROMERO NÚÑEZ, C. HEREDIA, R. Early onset canine generalized demodicosis. *Vet Dermatol*, 2017.

GORTEL, K. Recognizing pyoderma: more difficult than it may seem. *Vet Clin North Am Small Anim Pract*, 2013; 43(1):1–18.

MILLER, W. H., GRIFFIN, C. E., CAMPBELL, K. L. *Muller and Kirk's Small Animal Dermatology*, 7th ed, 2013. Elsevier Health Sciences.

## Chapter 3

GORTEL, K. Recognizing pyoderma: more difficult than it may seem. *Vet Clin North Am Small Anim Pract*, 2013; 43(1):1–18.

ALBANESE, F. *Atlas of dermatological cytology of dogs and cats*, 2010. Milan (Italy), Merial.

JANG, S. S., HIRSH, D. C. Rapidly growing members of the genus *Mycobacterium* affecting dogs and cats. *J Am Anim Hosp Assoc*, 2002; 38(3): 17–220.

MILLER, W. H., GRIFFIN, C. E., CAMPBELL, K. L. *Muller and Kirk's Small Animal Dermatology*, 7th ed, 2013. Elsevier Health Sciences.

## Chapter 4

GORTEL, K. Recognizing pyoderma: more difficult than it may seem. *Vet Clin Small Anim Pract*, 2013; 43(1):1–18.

GROSS, T. L., IHRKE, P. J., WALDER, E. J., AFFOLTER, V. K. *Skin diseases of the dog and cat: clinical and histopathologic diagnosis*, 2008. John Wiley & Sons.

MILLER, W. H., GRIFFIN, C. E., CAMPBELL, K. L. *Muller and Kirk's Small Animal Dermatology*, 7th ed, 2013. Elsevier Health Sciences.

PATERSON, S. Intertrigo in the dog: aetiology, clinical signs and therapy. *Comp Anim*, 2017; 22(2):72–77.

REIMANN, K. A., EVANS, M. G., CHALIFOUX, L. V. et al. Clinicopathologic characterization of canine juvenile celullitis. *Vet Pathol*, 1989; 26(6):499–504.

SCARFF, D. Intertrigo: the hidden face of canine atopic dermatitis. *Comp Anim*, 2016; 21(7):384–390.

## Chapter 5

ANDREWS, J. M. Determination of minimum inhibitory concentrations. *J Antimicrob Chemother*, 2001; 48(1):5–16.

ELNER, P. D., NEU, H. C. A method for interpreting minimum inhibitory concentration data. *J Am Med Assoc*, 1981; 246:1575–1578.

HILLIER, A., LLOYD, D. H., WEESE, J. S. et al. Guidelines for the diagnosis and antimicrobial therapy of canine superficial bacterial folliculitis (Antimicrobial Guidelines Working Group of the International Society for Companion Animal Infectious Diseases). *Vet Dermatol*, 2014.

LAMBERT, R. J. W., PEARSON, J. Susceptibility testing: accurate and reproducible minimum inhibitory concentration (MIC) and non-inhibitory concentration (NIC) values. *J Appl Microbiol*, 2000; 88(5):784–790.

MACGOWAN, A. P., WISE, R. Establishing MIC breakpoints and the interpretation of in vitro susceptibility tests. *J Antimicrob Chemother*, 2001; 48(1):17–28.

TURNIDGE, J., PATERSON, D. L. Setting and revising antibacterial susceptibility breakpoints. *Clin Microbiol Rev*, 2007; 20(3): 391–408.

VAUGHAN, D.F., LEMARIE, S.L. Comparison of culture and susceptibility results of superficial vs. biopsy specimens in dogs with superficial pyoderma. *Vet Dermatol*, 2008; 19(2):106–113.

WHITE, S. D., BROWN, A. E., CHAPMAN, P. L. et al. Evaluation of aerobic bacteriologic culture of epidermal collarette specimens in dogs with superficial pyoderma. *J Am Vet Med Assoc*, 2005; 226(6):904–908.

## Chapter 6

BANOVIC, F., OLIVRY, T., BÄUMER, W. et al. Diluted sodium hypochlorite (bleach) in dogs: antiseptic efficacy, local tolerability and in vitro effect on skin barrier function and inflammation. *Vet Dermatol*, 2018; 29(1):6–e5.

BORIO, S., COLOMBO, S., LA ROSA, G. et al. Effectiveness of a combined (4% chlorhexidine digluconate shampoo and solution) protocol in MRS and non-MRS canine superficial pyoderma: a randomized, blinded, antibiotic-controlled study. *Vet Dermatol*, 2015; 26(5):339–e72.

CLARK, S. M., LOEFFLER, A., BOND, R. Susceptibility in vitro of canine methicillin-resistant and-susceptible staphylococcal isolates to fusidic acid, chlorhexidine and miconazole: opportunities for topical therapy of canine superficial pyoderma. *J Antimicrob Chemother*, 2015; 70(7):2048–2052.

Frosini, S. M., Bond, R. Activity In Vitro of Clotrimazole against Canine Methicillin-Resistant and Susceptible Staphylococcus pseudintermedius. *Antibiotics*, 2017; 6(4):29.

Jeffers, J. G. Topical therapy for drug-resistant pyoderma in small animals. *Vet Clin Small Anim Pract*, 2013; 43(1):41–50.

Loeffler, A., Cobb, M. A., Bond, R. Comparison of a chlorhexidine and a benzoyl peroxide shampoo as sole treatment in canine superficial pyoderma. *Vet Rec*, 2011; 169(10):249–249.

Miller, W. H., Griffin, C. E., Campbell, K. L. *Muller and Kirk's Small Animal Dermatology*, 7th ed, 2013. Elsevier Health Sciences.

Mueller, R. S., Bergvall, K., Bensignor, E., Bond, R. A review of topical therapy for skin infections with bacteria and yeast. *Vet Dermatol*, 2012; 23(4):330–341.

Murayama, N., Terada, Y., Okuaki, M., Nagata, M. Dose assessment of 2% chlorhexidine acetate for canine superficial pyoderma. *Vet Dermatol*, 2011; 22(5):449–453.

## Chapter 7

Beco, L., Guaguère, E., Méndez, C. L. et al. Suggested guidelines for using systemic antimicrobials in bacterial skin infections: part 1—diagnosis based on clinical presentation, cytology and culture. *Vet Rec*, 2013; 172(3):72.

Beco, L., Guaguère, E., Méndez, C. L. et al. Suggested guidelines for using systemic antimicrobials in bacterial skin infections: part 2—antimicrobial choice, treatment regimens and compliance. *Vet Rec*, 2013; 172(6):156.

Hillier, A., Lloyd, D. H., Weese, J. S. et al. Guidelines for the diagnosis and antimicrobial therapy of canine superficial bacterial folliculitis (Antimicrobial Guidelines Working Group of the International Society for Companion Animal Infectious Diseases). *Vet Dermatol*, 2014.

Koch, S. N., Torres, S. M. F., Plumb, D. C. *Canine and feline dermatology drug handbook*, 2012. John Wiley & Sons.

Loeffler, A., Lloyd, D. H. What has changed in canine pyoderma? A narrative review. *Vet J*, 2018; 235:73–82.

Miller, W. H., Griffin, C. E., Campbell, K. L. *Muller and Kirk's Small Animal Dermatology*, 7th ed, 2013. Elsevier Health Sciences, pp. 200–207.

## Chapter 8

Frank, L. A., Loeffler, A. Meticillin-resistant *Staphylococcus pseudintermedius*: clinical challenge and treatment options. *Vet Dermatol*, 2012; 23(4):283–e56.

Julian, T., Singh, A., Rousseau, J., Weese, J. S. Methicillin-resistant staphylococcal contamination of cellular phones of personnel in a veterinary teaching hospital. *BMC research notes*, 2012; 5(1):193.

Loeffler, A., Lloyd, D. H. What has changed in canine pyoderma? A narrative review. *Vet J*, 2018; 235:73–82.

Pires dos Santos, T., Damborg, P., Moodley, A., Guardabassi, L. Systematic review on global epidemiology of methicillin-resistant *Staphylococcus pseudintermedius*: inference of population structure from multilocus sequence typing data. *Front Microbiol*, 2016; 7:1.599.

Singh, A., Walker, M., Rousseau, J., Monteith, G. J., Weese, J. S. Methicillin-resistant staphylococcal contamination of clothing worn by personnel in a veterinary teaching hospital. *Vet Surg*, 2013; 42(6):643–648.

Stefanetti, V., Bietta, A., Pascucci, L., et al. Investigation of the antibiotic resistance and biofilm formation of *Staphylococcus pseudintermedius* strains isolated from canine pyoderma. *Veterinaria italiana*, 2017; 53(4):289–296.

Worthing, K. A., Brown, J., Gerber, L. et al. Molecular epidemiology of methicillin-resistant staphylococci amongst veterinary personnel, personnel-owned pets, patients and the hospital environment of two companion animal veterinary hospitals. *Vet Microbiol*, 2018, 223:79–85.